"The End of All Diseases"

An Obscure San Diego Genius Develops A Cure For Cancer In 1930

*Based on the work and life of
inventor Royal Rife*

BY

R.E. PAYNE

ISBN: 1-4107-5342-5 (e-book)
ISBN: 1-4107-5340-9 (Paperback)
ISBN: 1-4107-5341-7 (Dust Jacket)

Library of Congress Control Number: 2003093252

This book is printed on acid free paper.

Printed in the United States of America
Bloomington, IN

1stBooks - rev. 06/26/03

DEDICATION

Steve Howell for research assistance

Chinese Historical Society of Greater San Diego and Baja California

Maria Arroyo Prokop for assistance in retrieving priceless newspaper

stories about Rife

"For our wrestling is not against

flesh and blood;

but against principalities

and powers,

against the rulers of the world

of this darkness,

against the spirits of wickedness

in the high places."

(Ephesians 6, 12)

1

In every generation men and women arise who perform near miracles for a time and then are lost to history. In 1931, 44 of the most respected medical authorities in North America honored such a man-a scientist-at a banquet billed as "The End of All Diseases." A few years later, the Medical Research Committee of the University of Southern California, comprising five physicians and a pathologist, treated 16 cancer patients from the Pasadena General Hospital, all considered incurable, with a device that identifies and destroys any virus or bacteria. Fourteen of the 16 patients are declared clinically cured in less than three months. After adjusting treatment, the other two patients are also cured over the next few weeks. The San Diego scientist is Royal Rife and his "electronic antibiotic" is known as the Frequency Generator.

Rife invented the most powerful microscope of his time to chase his conviction that a cure for diseases cannot be found until the live viruses causing the disease are visible to the human eye. The Rife microscope weighed over 200 pounds and consisted of about 6,000 moving parts. As early as 1930, Rife was looking into live diseased organisms through his microscope, an unparalleled break-through made possible only by his invention. Rife later used his Frequency Generator to irradiate these diseased organisms until he exposed the frequency rate that causes them to explode, as does glass shatter when the right frequency is reached. In more than 400 animal tests Rife found that by bombarding the diseased organisms, he killed them, rendering them unable to cause disease in the body of the animals tested. Diseases cured harmlessly and without drugs!

Rife's primary financial backer was his father-in-law, Ah Quin, the most successful Chinese businessman of the period in San Diego. Quin idolized his daughter Maime and he believed in Rife and his work. He gave generously, frequently tapping into his wealth to provide the laboratory and instruments required for research, and to provide Maime and her husband with a very comfortable lifestyle. Through the powers of personality and intelligence, Quin successfully bridged the social gap between the Chinese and the white power structure of his day. Quin introduced important and wealthy persons to Rife, who were easily influenced by Quin to join him in bankrolling Rife and his project.

Quin's first venture in San Diego was successful, a retail business specializing in Chinese imported stock that attracted clientele from both the Chinese and American communities, but he was also known for selling unusual items, like birds. He expanded so quickly he moved into larger quarters. During this period he came into contact with many powerful persons, notably, Frank Kimball. Kimball, the founder of National City, helped convince the Atchison, Topeka, and Santa Fe Railroad to add a connection to National City. On October 12, 1880, the California Southern Railroad was chartered. The line would run from National City through San Diego, and up the coast as far as Santa Barbara, more than 100 miles. A year later, it was decided to hook up with the Atlantic and Pacific Railroad near Barstow, adding another 80 miles. But in order to do this, more and better labor was needed. This is where Ah Quin stepped in and made his reputation.

He sold his ideal of using Chinese labor to build the railroads. Quin recruited this labor. Soon nearly 100 Chinese arrived on the Senator, a steamship, and the local paper carried the announcement of the arrivals. Quin succeeded in placing all of the laborers, although there were some contractors who refused to hire them. Quin controlled many of the logistics involving the Chinese laborers, including the supplying of the food and other needs. The Chinese lived in camps under tents and Quin furnished them with the food they knew: fish, tea, and rice. Quin made money on every aspect of the operation; he soon became quite wealthy. He was actively engaged in railroad building until at least 1885.

In the meantime, Quin's retail business profited enormously from his other efforts and his real estate holdings continued to swell, including farming and food distribution. Quin's wealth made it possible for Rife to spend all of his time on his inventions, and his dream of identifying and, possibly, curing diseases without drugs.

———

The specialists of the University of Southern California that evaluated the therapy provided by Rife in his laboratory of the tests conducted by the Medical Research Committee are: Rufus Klein-Schmidt, president, University of Southern California; Milbank Johnson, president, Southern California American Medical Association (AMA); Arthur Kendall, director, Northwestern University Medical School; Edward Kopps, Metabolic Clinic, La Jolla; George Fische, Children's Hospital, NYC; Karl Meyer, Hooper Foundation, San Francisco; Whaler Morrison, chief surgeon, Santa Fe Railway; and George Dock.

In Rife's own words: "We succeeded with the Frequency Generator. I actually discovered the lethal frequency for a number of different organisms, which blew them up, killing them. For example, Typhoid 1.5-1.6 KHz; E-coli 799-804 HZ; TB 1.5-16 KHz; Pneumonia 770-780 Hz; and Staphylococcus 725-730 Hz."

"All of the cancer patients tested at my lab under the auspices of USC are cured."

So, why aren't doctors using it? If the Rife invention achieved everything it was supposed to do, and if the Frequency Generator did cure cancer, why are doctors not using this therapy? Why did they not even get a chance to use it? Why were assurances of government-funded laboratory testing not kept?

Physicians who were using the Rife methods were coerced into ditching them by the AMA. Reports of authentic cures were denied publicity in the AMA Journal, so it is unlikely very many doctors ever heard of Rife or his microscope or Frequency Generator. Without the backing and publicity generally provided by the AMA, it was out of the question for independent laboratories to carry out testing.

Now begins the story of how the pharmaceutical cartel, hospitals, the autocratic leader of the AMA, the government and a handful of other special interests preclude the Rife device from being accepted for further testing by the approved United States Government laboratories, an indispensable requisite for verification, and use as a treatment for cancer. Rife's opponents, especially that of the AMA, all use deception, intimidation, intrigue, perjury, treachery and other tools usually ascribed to lesser personages, to help the pharmaceutical cartel and others to ridicule Rife, without ever testing the Rife cure on patients.

More than money is implicated here. The issue was and remains nothing less than survival. Today we know that and much more. The AMA believes in bigness. The pharmaceutical cartel believes in drugs. The government believes in control.

And remember, the AMA has power over how medicine is taught and practiced.

Rife and his friends did not have blind faith in their capacity to find a cure for cancer or other diseases. They sought after and plead for independent, official testing. Rife repeatedly said that he understood that no new innovation was exempt from uncertainties, obstacles and risks. But Rife was a prisoner of a fate he could not alter or escape. He ended up in total conflict with an Establishment he did not comprehend.

Disease is profitable. Any new technology that eliminates disease without drugs threatens the loss of several billion dollars a week to the pharmaceutical cartel. And what about the grants to researchers, universities, hospitals and others? Who or what could approve of eliminating this? Let's not forget, but the health care industry itself— the entire industry, including insurance—would dry up and go away, if there was a cure for diseases that did not involve physicians, hospitals and drugs.

———

Royal Rife was born in Nebraska in 1888 and died in San Diego in 1971. During his life, the disease of cancer increased from only 1 in 25 to 1 in 3 persons. During this period, he watched the American Cancer Society become a household name, collecting hundreds of millions of dollars for a disease that was possibly cured by Rife in his laboratories in the 1930's. Rife also witnessed the approval by the FDA of cancer drugs, some of which had mortality rates of nearly 20 percent. With such drugs it was a matter of time whether the patient died from the drug or the disease. Today it is projected it cost about $400,000 to treat a single cancer patient.

The physicians who actually witnessed the successful therapy offered by Rife's technology either lost their foundation grants and or were in danger of loss of hospital privileges. Some others received mysterious rewards. Dr. Arthur Kendall, for example, reportedly retired during the Depression after receiving a payment of $200,000 or more. Dr. George Dock received a huge grant and then quickly disavowed his association with Rife.

Rife was betrayed for greed and money. Regrettably, Rife was dealt a fatal blow by the system and others who dreaded victory for a scientist—instead of a medical doctor—especially one who effectively challenged the pharmaceutical-medical industries. Rife spent most of his adult life in research and in the process cataloged volumes of work, including film and photography, as well as voice recorded records. He encountered unexplained disappearances of research data over a period of time from his laboratory, including many of his written records, engineering and other technical drawings. No one was ever caught.

During an age where computers were not in common use and copying of documents was laborious, if not impossible, Rife found it tough to replace his losses. Worst, he did not know who was to fault. Just when things were bad, they got worse: someone broke into his laboratory and stole what they thought was a complete Universal microscope. Actually, the microscope was not fully assembled. What they got was approximately 5,000 parts of the 6,000-piece instrument.

Rife hired additional employees who also worked for the house as culinary or housekeeping help; he assigned them the extra duty of surveillance over the laboratory when he was not there. He later alleged that it was one or more of these employees who may have been involved in the stealing, but his associates questioned this, as the employees had no apparent motive to steal research data or scientific instruments. Nor did they understand or know what it was Rife was researching.

Rife did not agree with the idea of a conspiracy to prevent his further progress with technology and research to cure diseases without drugs. But an incident in New Jersey made him skeptical. One of his Frequency Generators was being tested by an independent laboratory, and just as they were due to release a report on its effectiveness, the Burnett Lab was ruined in a multi-million dollar fire that was later suspected as arson. The laboratory had advised Rife that they were going to corroborate the same positive outcomes he had reported. The magnitude of this autonomous substantiation cannot be overstated. Rife believed it was going to open closed minds and doors and create pressure for AMA attention.

The method of treatment advocated by Rife, a nontoxic alternative to drugs, conflicted with the authorities that controlled the pharmaceutical and medical industries. He and his colleagues, those medical doctors who had been using his Frequency Generator with success, were deprived of access to the system they required to find out the ultimate use of the Frequency Generator in established medicine. One can only hypothesize now on what could have happened, if the process had worked and generations of sincere scientists and doctors had been permitted to refine Rife's invention.

The final blow fell when the company that manufactured the Frequency Generator came under the legal assault of agents for the pharmaceutical industry. The company could not sustain the legal expenses during the Depression and commercial production of Rife's instruments ended. One ought to conclude that the labor of a lifetime resulted in very little, if any, good; and that whatever positive results may have been possible, they died with Rife.

The use of Rife's Frequency Generator was barred by 1939, the instruments all confiscated by authorities from the clinics where they were in use in California. Rife was forced into court. Rife's microscope and Frequency Generator had just accomplished successfully isolating TB, Polio, cancer and other diseases and when turned to the correct frequency for each one, the diseased organisms were destroyed, according to his records.

"Having spent every dime I earned in my research for the benefit of mankind, I have ended up a pauper, but I achieved the impossible and would do it again," he wrote in a court affidavit.

While Rife had lived a comfortable, even extravagant life-style, thanks to his father-in-law and wife, even having the privilege of owning a couple of Rolls Royce automobiles, his life sped out of control as he became addicted to both alcohol and valium, perhaps drowning himself in self-pity. It was a phenomenon he lived to the age of 83, dying in a nursing home.

But did Rife's secrets die with him?

2

"The doctors told my mother the spinal cord injury I suffered would leave me unable to ever walk again. No one informed me. I was only 12 years old. It never really occurred to me that my volleyball days were over or that I would be lucky to be restricted to a wheelchair the rest of my life. I was a girl who breathed to play sports and swim. I had already made up my mind that I wanted to try for a college scholarship in swimming. I was winning every meet I entered," she said, flipping through a photo album, occasionally pointing out a photo of herself swimming or playing volleyball or twirling a baton in a parade.

Anjanette de la Houssaye, now 31, spoke without regret; her courage greatly admired by Howard Horowitz, a producer of TV movies based on real life experiences. If he was looking for a real-life story about a woman with courage, he found one. "Does it trouble you to talk about this?"

"Not at all. I do it as much as I can. I am frequently requested by various organizations to tell my story. It lifts their hopes. A person in such a predicament needs hope. If I can lend a hand to give others courage to go on with their lives, then I know I am giving a positive outcome to what happened to me."

But Anjanette was not always positive. "I cried for hours at a time. I was lonely; I felt isolated and useless. I woke up one day to see my world turned upside down. I did not comprehend why God allowed this to happen to me. I loved God. I was a devoted churchgoer. I sang in the choir. I volunteered. I was bitter and hateful to those who loved me."

"Well, when was the moment of change? The time when all that left and the positive attitude kicked in?"

"The pastor of my church came by with a room full of the congregation. He said that God did love me, and that I needed my faith more then ever. He and my mother held my hands while other members of my congregation touched my hair, arms, body and legs. He prayed and we prayed and when it was over, I felt like a boulder had been removed from my shoulders. All of a sudden, I knew that if I was going to get better, that I had to accept what happened."

"You realized a new reason for your life?"

"I did. My mom told me stories about her older brother, my Uncle Moreau, who was an engineer who lived at Prince Edward Island. He always had an opportunistic outlook, apparently devoting himself to working on an important medical device, sacrificing everything so that he could devote his time and talents to this long-standing venture in San Diego. I hope to discover that one motivating thing that I want to do that will occupy my talents and efforts for the rest of my life. For a while, I thought journalism was it, but after several years in the newspaper industry, I must admit it does not measure up."

"Maybe you need to write a book."

"Maybe."

"What happened to your Uncle Moreau?"

"We really do not know. He died and since my mother is deceased, he left everything he had to me. So far as I know, all he has is an old house that has rooms rented in it. From what the attorneys tell me, he was living on rental income, and a small pension from the government."

"Your inheritance?"

"Yes, and I must go to PEI next month to sign all the documents and reach a decision what to do with the rooming house. I was born in New Brunswick but we left when I was a child. I never visited PEI. I am looking forward to getting away from British Columbia. Actually, I am taking a leave of absence from the paper."

"Prince Edward Island-the hone of Anne of Green Gables!"

"Yes, of course. I grew up on Cape Tormentine on the extreme southeast corner of New Brunswick. We lived in a big but old house that overlooked the Northumberland Strait to the north. I still feel the stiff, cold winds even now just talking about it," she grimaced. "My dad was a lobsterman who died young in an accident. My mother had

13

few business skills, but she turned our home into a bed and breakfast to increase our income. We only had three rooms to rent and renters were hard to find except when construction was underway. Mom also cooked lobsters by order, but we barely squeezed out a living. She sold the house to the province, so we relocated to British Columbia."

"I find that story irresistible. I am visualizing the setting already. Please let me know how you turn out with your adventure to PEI and your inheritance. It may become part of our story for the movie-"

"-Oh, no, what adventure? I am flying into St. Johns and renting a van. I don't know what I will do with the rooming house at PEI, except hope that it produces enough income for me to take some time off from working! I do not think it will be very adventuresome."

"Maybe. May I ask a very personal question?"

"Of course. I better answer!"

"You are a beautiful woman. Being in the TV movie business, I tend to cast roles all the time. Upon first seeing you, I thought immediately of Madeline Stowe but now, I am prone to think of...I better not get into this-"

"Excellent! Leave it at that—how can I improve on that selection? Anyway, go ahead, I have a hunch you were going to inquire about my love life."

"Do you mind? I don't want you imagining sex is what I am interested in -"

"-My love life? No, I don't mind talking about it, as it is a matter of curiosity to both men and women. Can I have sex? Do I feel it?

Can I move? I've heard them all. If I am optioning my story to you, I should expect to answer questions. First, I do not have a boy friend or a steady date at this time, but I have had in the past. Actually, quite a few, even with the wheelchair and crutches in college. Truthfully, young men in college did not seem to even notice those aids. They supposed it was a temporary condition or the result of a recent accident or something like that," she said, spreading her shoulder length hair back behind her ears. "Because of all the rehabbing, I guess my body toned up. Candidly, as a small town newspaper editor, there are few opportunities to meet new men, and it is not something I reflect about very often. If and when I meet up with the right person, I am praying that I have the good judgment to know who it is!"

Paralyzed from a swimming accident, Anjanette was lucky. Following years of rehabilitation she walked with crutches, only occasionally requiring a wheelchair for long strolls through mega shopping malls or 'walks' in the park, or for using in wheelchair marathons or other sporting events. She drives a van with special hand controls. "I was fortunate I did not have a more severe injury, like actor Christopher Reeve. I am advised that every spinal chord injury is different. I actually regained about 50 percent of the strength in my hands and some movement of my fingers. I am able to use a regular computer, if I have to—to some extant. I think I am a very blessed person."

A blessed person, perhaps, but at periods, still, a very frustrated one, vacillating from emotional highs to feeling overwhelmed and

15

burdened. "I am frustrated but not from lack of sex. I regret that I have not yet found my calling in life. I am disappointed it is not journalism. I was certain when I was young that it was." She had no new dreams to chase, but was grateful for the opportunity to sell her life story and to see it produced as a TV movie. She sought more from life than getting along and conquering her handicap. She often thought of Uncle Moreau, or at least the way he was described to her by her mom. She envied him. Although his life was apparently not successful financially, he believed in something so strongly that he sacrificed everything to be involved in it. Anjanette longed for this.

As recently as a couple of years ago she wanted her own Christian ministry. She prayed about it with friends, but realized that her judgment was clouded by her accident, and resulting lack of life experience in the real world. Covering city council meetings in a Canadian town of only 8,000 population does not offer too many worldly opportunities. Although she had traveled to the United States to visit several states when she was in college, she did not feel worldly. Also, her relationships experience with men was minimal; she unquestionably did not feel qualified to give advice on the subject of relationships or love.

There was a man who meant something to her but that was five or more years ago. A physical therapist that had seen, held and rubbed virtually every part of her body at one time or another. A big man, but a gentle one. She looked forward to therapy with him-his name was Theodore Washington, but she called him Ted. He was from

Louisiana but he grew up in Spokane, Washington. He was about ten years older but that didn't matter. What did matter is that he was an avowed agnostic and African-American. Ted said his surname was not in honor of George Washington, that his family accepted the name generations ago as slaves in Washington Parish where they toiled on cotton fields.

Ted was the first non-white person she had ever really known beyond a chance hello at class or the office. She thought he had very deep but unexpressed feelings for her, and no matter what she did or said to encourage him, he remained professionally detached. She thought it was shyness. She knew it had nothing to do with her disability as she had worked with Ted for years in rehab; he had a special heart for helping those who needed it. Unable to continue concealing her feelings for Ted, she told him.

Ted did not believe in 'mixed' marriage, he said, and he did not want any other kind of relationship with "Anjie", as he called her. His mixing concern was religious, not racial. He said he did not want to spend the rest of his life being preached to by a 'born-again, spirit filled Christian'. He loved her and always would. He said so, but not in so many words. He arranged for a new therapist and refused to take her calls. Anjie cried for weeks.

When Horowitz left, he promised that a contract to option her life story would be in the mail soon. "I know you hear about the big million dollar deals in the media but believe me, this is not the type of story that brings big money. You have to be on the front page for that.

But this will pay you US$50,000, and all you have to do is sign the option and hope we sell it to a network."

She agreed. With the $50,000 from Horowitz and the income from the rooming house in PEI, she may become independent enough to write that book.

3

Royal Rife had one of the best-equipped laboratories in the world. In the basement, he had facilities for as many as 1,000 animals. He had a surgical room for animals with sterilizers of the steam type, and a pathology room complete with microscopes of all types including virus microscopes, which he had designed and built for isolation of cancer virus, TB virus, typhoid virus and many other viruses. His research laboratory was air-conditioned and humidity controlled to one tenth of a degree. He had a stop motion microscope set up for the life study of microorganisms from the cradle to the grave. The laboratory also had a million volt X-Ray, frequency instruments, electronic test equipment, precision lathes, mills, drill presses, and all equipment necessary to make instruments, microscopes, and glass blowing.

Royal Rife invented the system of killing or de-activating pathogenic organisms by electronic waves or frequencies produced by instruments that he invented. He began his experimental work as early as 1915. By 1920 his theory developed. In the process he had studied such pathogenic organisms as tetanus, typhoid, gonorrhea, syphilis, staphylococci, pneumonia, strertothrix, streptococci, tuberculosis, sarcoma, carcinoma, leprosy, polio, cholera, actinomycosis, glanders, bubonic plague, anthrax, influenza, herpes, cataracts, glaucomia, colitis, sinus, ulcers and many other virus bacteria and fungi. Rife obtained these organisms from the Mayo Clinic, Northwestern Medical University in Chicago, the Paradise Valley Sanatorium and the Hooper Foundation.

He had to invent a microscope to do this research. The Smithsonian Institute released a report on Rife's Universal Microscope in 1944 in the Journal of the Franklin Institute. Here are excerpts from this report.

"It is only a reasonable supposition, but already, in one instance, a very successful and highly commendable achievement on the part of Dr. Royal Raymond Rife of San Diego, California, who, for many years, has built and worked with light microscopes which far surpass the theoretical limitations of the ordinary variety of instrument, all the Rife scopes possessing superior ability to attain high magnification with accompanying high resolution.

"The largest and most powerful of these, the Universal Microscope, developed in 1933, consists of 5,682 parts and is so called because of its adaptability in all fields of microscopical work, being fully equipped with separate substage condenser units for transmitted and monochromatic beam dark-field, polarized, and slit-ultra illumination, including also a special device for crystallography. The entire optical system of lenses and prisms as well as the illuminating units are made of block-crystal quartz, quartz being especially transparent to ultraviolet radiations.

"This illuminating unit used for examining the filterable forms of disease organisms contains 14 lenses and prisms, 3 of which are in the high-intensity incandescent lamp, 4 in the Risley prism, and 7 in the achromatic condenser which, incidentally, has a numerical aperture of 1.40. Between the source of light and the specimen are subtended two circular, wedge-shaped, block-crystal quartz prisms for the purpose of polarizing the light passing through the specimen, polarization being the practical application of the theory that light waves vibrate in all planes perpendicular to the direction in which they are propagated.

"Therefore, when light comes into contact with a polarizing prism, it is divided or split into two beams, one of which is refracted to such an extent that it is reflected to the side of the prism without, of course, passing through the prism while the second ray, bent considerably less, is thus enabled to pass through the prism to illuminate the specimen.

"When the quartz prisms on the universal microscope, which may be rotated with vernier control through 360 degrees, are rotated in opposite directions, they serve to bend the transmitted beams of light at variable angles of incidence while, at the same time, a spectrum is projected up into the axis of the microscope, or rather a small portion of the spectrum to the other, going all the way from the infrared to the ultraviolet.

"Now, when that portion of the spectrum is reached in which both the organism and the color band vibrate in exact accord, one with the other, a definite characteristic spectrum is emitted by the organism. In the case of the filter-passing form of the Bacillus Typhosus, for instance, a blue spectrum is emitted and the plane of polarization deviated plus (+) 4.8 degrees.

"The predominating chemical constituents of the organism are next ascertained after which the quartz prisms are adjusted or set, by means of vernier control, to minus (-) 4.8 degrees (again in the case of the filter-passing form of the Bacillus Typhosus) so that the opposite angle of refraction may be obtained.

"A monochromatic beam of light, corresponding exactly to the frequency of the organism (for Dr. Rife has found that each disease organism responds to and has a definite wave length, a fact confirmed by British medical research workers) is then sent up through the specimen and the direct transmitted light, thus enabling the observer to view the organism stained in its true chemical color and revealing its own individual structure in a field which is brilliant with light.

"The objectives used on the universal microscope are a 1.12 dry lens, a 1.16 water immersion, a 1.18 oil immersion, and a 1.25 oil immersion. The rays of light refracted by the specimen enter the objective and are then carried up the tube in parallel rays through 21 light bends to the ocular, a tolerance of less than one wave length of visible light only being permitted in the core beam, or chief ray, of illumination.

"Now, instead of the light rays starting up the tube in a parallel fashion, tending to converge as they rise higher and finally crossing each other, arriving at the ocular separated by considerable distance as would be the case with an ordinary microscope, in the universal tube the rays also start their rise parallel to each other but, just as they are about to pull them out parallel again, another prism being inserted each time the rays are about ready to cross.

"These prisms, inserted in the tube, which are adjusted and held in alignment by micrometer screws of 100 threads to the inch in special tracks made of magnelium (magnelium having the closest coefficient of expansion of any metal to quartz), are separated by a distance of only 30 millimeters.

"Thus, the greatest distance that the image in the universal microscope is projected through any one media, either quartz or air, is 30 millimeters instead of the 160, 180, or 190 millimeters as in the empty or air-filled tubes of an ordinary microscope, the total distance which the light rays travel zigzag fashion through the universal tube being 449 millimeters, although the physical length of the tube itself is 229 millimeters.

"It will be recalled that if one pierces a black strip of paper or cardboard with the point of a needle and then brings the card up close to the eye so that the hole is in the optic axis, a small brilliantly lighted object will appear larger and clearer, revealing more fine detail, than if it were viewed from the same distance without the assistance of the card.

"This is explained by the fact that the beam of light passing through the card is very narrow, the rays entering the eye, therefore, being practically parallel, whereas without the card the beam of light is much wider and the diffusion circles much larger. It is this principle of parallel rays in the universal microscope and the resultant shortening of projection distance between any two blocks or prisms plus the fact that objectives can thus be substituted for oculars, these "oculars" being three matched pairs of 10 millimeter, 7 millimeter, and 4 millimeter objectives in short mounts, which would make possible not only the unusually high magnification and resolution but which serve to eliminate all distortion as well as all chromatic and spherical aberration.

"Quartz slides with especially thin quartz cover glasses are used when a tissue section or culture slant is examined, the tissue section itself also being very thin. An additional observational tube and ocular which yield a magnification of 1,800 diameters are provided so that that portion of the specimen which is desired to be examined may be located so that the observer can adjust himself more readily when viewing a section at a high magnification.

"The universal stage is a double rotating stage graduated through 360 degrees in quarter-minute arc divisions, the upper segment carrying the mechanical stage having a movement of 40 degrees, plus or minus. Heavily constructed joints and screw adjustments maintain rigidity of the microscope which weighs 200 pounds and stands 24 inches high, the bases of the scope being nickel cast-steel plates, accurately surfaced, and equipped with three leveling screws and two spirit levels set at angles of 90 degrees. The coarse adjustment, a block thread screw with 40 threads to the inch, slides in a 1 1/2 dovetail, which gibes directly onto the pillar post. The weight of the quadruple nosepiece and the objective system is taken care of by the intermediate adjustment at the top of the body tube. The stage, in conjunction with a hydraulic lift, acts as a lever in operating the fine adjustment.

"A 6-gauge screw having 100 threads to the inch is worked through a gland into a hollow, glycerine-filled post, the glycerine being displaced and replaced at will as the screw is turned clockwise or anticlockwise, allowing a 5-to-1 ratio on the lead screw. This, accordingly, assures complete absence of drag and inertia. The fine adjustment being 700 times more sensitive then that of ordinary microscopes, the length of time required to focus the universal ranges up to 1 1/2 hours which, while on first consideration, may seem a disadvantage, is after all but a slight inconvenience when compared with the many years of research and the hundreds of thousands of dollars spent and being spent in an effort to isolate and to look upon disease-causing organisms in their true form.

"Working together back in 1931 and using one of the smaller Rife microscope having a magnification and resolution of 17,000 diameters, Dr. Rife and Dr. Arthur Isaac Kendall, of the department of bacteriology of Northwestern University Medical School, were able to observe and demonstrate the presence of the filter-passing forms of Bacillus Typhosus. An agar slant culture of the Rawlings strain of Bacillus Typhosus was first prepared by Dr. Kendall and inoculated into 6 cc of "Kendall" K Medium, a medium rich in protein but poor in peptone and consisting of 100 mg. of dried hog intestine and 6 cc of tyrode solution (containing neither glucose nor glycerine) which mixture is shaken well so as to moisten the dried intestine powder and then sterilized in the autoclave, 15 pounds for 15 minutes, alterations of the medium being frequently necessary depending upon the requirements for different organisms.

"Now, after a period of 18 hours in this K Medium, the culture was passed through a Berkefeld "N" filter, a drop of the filtrate being added to another 6 cc. of K Medium and incubated at 37 degrees C. Forty-eight hours later this same process was repeated, the "N" filter again being used, after which it was noted that the culture no longer responded to peptone medium, growing now only in the protein medium. When again, within 24 hours, the culture was passed through a filter-the finest Berkefeld "W" filter, a drop of the filtrate was once more added to 6 cc. of K Medium and incubated at 37 degrees c., a period of 3 days elapsing before a new culture was transferred to K Medium and yet another 3 days before a new culture was prepared. Then, viewed under an ordinary microscope, these cultures were observed to be turbid and to reveal no bacilli whatsoever. When viewed by means of dark-field illumination and oil-immersion lens, however, the presence of small, actively motile granules was established, although nothing at all of their individual structure could be ascertained. Another period of 4 days was allowed to elapse before these cultures were transferred to K Medium and incubated at 37 degrees C for 24 hours when they were then examined under the Rife microscope where, as was mentioned earlier, the filterable typhoid bacilli, emitting a blue spectrum, caused the plane of polarization to be deviated plus 4.8 degrees.

"Then when the opposite angle of refraction was obtained by means of adjusting the polarizing prisms to minus 4.8 degrees and the cultures illuminated by a monochromatic beam coordinated in frequency with the chemical constituents of the typhoid bacillus, small oval actively motile, bright turquoise-blue bodies were observed at a magnification of 5,000 diameters, in high contrast to the colorless and motionless debris of the medium. These observations were repeated eight times, the complete absence of these bodies in uninoculated control K Media also being noted.

"To further confirm their findings, Drs. Rife and Kendall next examined 18-hour-old cultures which had been inoculated into K Medium and incubated at 37 degrees C., since it is just at this stage of growth in this medium and at this temperature that the cultures become filterable. And, just as had been anticipated, ordinary dark-field examination revealed unchanged, long, actively motile bacilli; bacilli having granules within their substance; and free-swimming, actively motile granules; while under the Rife microscope were demonstrated the same long, unchanged, almost colorless bacilli; bacilli, practically colorless, inside and at one end of which was a turquoise-blue granule resembling the filterable forms of the typhoid bacillus; and free-swimming, small, oval, actively motile, turquoise-blue granules. By transplanting the cultures of the filter-passing organisms or virus into a broth, they were seen to change over again into their original rod like forms.

"At the same time that these findings of Drs. Rife and Kendall were confirmed by Dr. Edward C. Rosenow, of the Mayo Foundation, the magnification with accompanying resolution of 8,000 diameters of the Rife microscope, operated by Dr. Rife, was checked against a dark-field oil-immersion scope operated by Dr. Kendall and an ordinary 2-mm. oil-immersion objective, x 10 ocular, Zeiss scope operated by Dr. Rosenow at a magnification of 900 diameters. Examinations of gram and safranin-stained films of culture of Bacillus typhosus, gram and safranin-stained films of blood and of the sediment of the spinal fluid from a case of acute poliomyelitis were made with the result that bacilli, streptococci, erythrocytes, polymorphonuclear leukocytes, and lymphocytes measuring nine times the diameter of the same specimens observed under the Zeiss scope at a magnification and resolution of 900 diameters, were revealed with unusual clarity. Seen under the dark-field microscope were moving bodies presumed to be the filterable turquois-blue bodies of the typhoid bacillus which, as Dr. Rosenow has declared in his report (Observations on filter-passing forms of Eberthella-typhi-

Bacillus typhosus - and of the streptococcus from poliomyelitis, Proc. Staff Meeting Mayo Clinic, July 13, 1932), were so "unmistakably demonstrated" with Rife microscope, while under the Zeiss scope stained and hanging-drop preparations of clouded filtrate culture were found to be uniformly negative.

"With the Rife microscope also were demonstrated brownish-gray cocci and diplococci in hanging-drop preparations of the filtrates of streptococcus from poliomyelitis. These cocci and diplococci, similar in size and shape to those seen in the culture although of more uniform intensity, and characteristic of the medium in which they had been cultivated, were surrounded by a clear halo about twice the width of that at the margins of the debris and of the Bacillus typhosus. Stained films of filtrates and filtrate sediments examined under the Zeiss microscope, and hanging-drop, dark-field preparations revealed no organisms, however. Brownish-gray cocci and diplococci of the exact same size and density as those observed in the filtrates of the streptococcus cultures were also revealed in hanging-drop preparations of the virus of poliomyelitis underthe Rife microscope, while no organisms at all could be seen in either the stained films of filtrates and filtrate sediments examined with the Zeiss scope or in hanging-drop preparations examined by means of the dark-field. Again using the Rife microscope at a magnification of 8,000 diameters, numerous nonmotile cocci and diplococci of a bright-to-pale pink in color were seen in hanging-drop preparations of filtrates of Herpes encephalitic virus. Although these were observed to be

29

comparatively smaller then the cocci and diplococci of the streptococcus and poliomyelitis viruses, they were shown to be of fairly even density, size and form and surrounded by a halo.

"Again, both the dark-field and Zeiss scopes failed to reveal any organisms, and none of the three microscopes disclosed the presence of such diplococci in hanging-drop preparation of the filtrate of a normal rabbit brain. Dr. Rosenow has since revealed these organisms with the ordinary microscope at a magnification of 1,000 diameters by means of his special staining method and with the electron microscope at a magnification of 12,000 diameters. Dr. Rosenow has expressed the opinion that the inability to see these and other similarly revealed organisms is due, not necessarily to the minuteness of the organisms, but rather to the fact that they are of a nonstaining, hyaline structure. Results with the Rife microscopes, he thinks, are due to the "ingenious methods employed rather than to excessively high magnification." He has declared also, in the report mentioned previously, that "Examination under the Rife microscope of specimens containing objects visible with the ordinary microscope, leaves no doubt of the accurate visualization of objects or particulate matter by direct observation at the extremely high magnification obtained with this instrument."

"Exceedingly high powers of magnification with accompanying high powers of resolution may be realized with all of the Rife microscopes, one of which, having magnification and resolution up to 18,000 diameters, is now being used at the British School of Tropical

Medicine in England. In a recent demonstration of another of the smaller Rife scopes (May 16, 1942) before a group of doctors including Dr. J.H. Renner, of Santa Barbara, Calif.; Dr. Roger A. Schmidt, of San Francisco, Calif.; Dr. Lois Bronson Slade, of Alameda, Calif.; Dr. Lucile B. Larkin, of Bellingham, Wash.; Dr. E. F. Larkin, of Bellingham, Wash.; and Dr. W. J. Gier, of San Diego, Calif., a Zeiss ruled grading was examined, first under an ordinary commercial microscope equipped with a 1.8 high dry lens and X 10 ocular, and then under the Rife microscope. Whereas 50 lines were revealed with the commercial instrument and considerable aberration, both chromatic and spherical noted, only 5 lines were seen with the Rife scope, these 5 lines being so highly magnified that they occupied the entire field, without any aberration whatsoever being apparent. Dr. Renner, in a discussion of his observations, stated, "The entire field to its very edges and across the center had a uniform clearness that was not true on the conventional instrument." Following the examination of the grading, an ordinary unstained blood film was observed under the same two microscopes. In this instance, 100 cells were seen to spread throughout the field of the commercial instrument while but 10 cells filled the field of the Rife scope.

"The universal microscope, of course, is the most powerful Rife scope, possessing a resolution of 31,000 diameters and magnification of 60,000 diameters. With this it is possible to view the interior of the 'pin-point' cells, those cells situated between the normal tissue cells and just visible under the ordinary microscope, and to observe the smaller cells which compose the interior of these pin-point cells. When one of these smaller cells in magnified, still smaller cells are seen within its structure. And when one of the still smaller cells, in its turn, is magnified, it, too, is seen to be composed of smaller cells. Each of the 16 times this process of magnification and resolution can be repeated, it is demonstrated that there are smaller cells within the smaller cells, a fact which amply testifies as to the magnification and resolving power obtainable with the universal microscope.

"More then 20,000 laboratory cultures of carcinoma were grown and studied over a period of 7 years by Dr. Rife and his assistants in what, at the time, appeared to be a fruitless effort to isolate the filter-passing form, or virus, which Dr. Rife believed to be present in this condition. Then, in 1932, the reactions in growth of bacterial cultures to light from the rare gasses was observed, indicating a new approach to the problem. Accordingly, blocks of tissue one-half centimeter square, taken from an unulcerated breast carcinoma, were placed in a circular glass loop filled with argon gas to a pressure of 14 millimeters, and a current of 5,000 volts applied for 24 hours, after which the tubes were placed in a 2-inch water vacuum and incubated at 37 degrees C. for 24 hours. Using a specially designed 1.12 dry lens, equal in amplitude of magnification to the 2-mm. apochromatic oil-immersion lens, the cultures were then examined under the universal microscope, at a magnification of 10,000 diameters, where very much animated, purplish-red, filterable forms, measuring less then one-twentieth of a micron in dimension, were observed. Carried through 14 transplants from K Medium to K Medium, this B. X. virus remained constant; inoculated into 426 Albino rats, tumors "with all the true pathology of neoplastic tissue" were developed. Experiments conducted in the Rife Laboratories have established the fact that these characteristic diplococci are found in the blood monocytes in 92 percent of all cases of neoplastic diseases. It has also been demonstrated that the virus of cancer, like the viruses of other diseases, can be easily changed from one form to another by means of altering the media upon which it is grown. With the first change in media, the B. X. virus becomes considerably enlarged although its purplish-red color remains unchanged.

"Observation of the organism with an ordinary microscope is made possible by a second alteration of the media. A third change is undergone upon asparagus base media where the B. X. virus is transformed from its filterable state into cryptomyces pleomorphia fungi, these fungi being identical morphologically both microscopically to that of the orchid and of the mushroom. And yet a fourth change may be said to take place when this cryptomyces pleomorphia, permitted to stand as a stock culture for the period of metastasis, becomes the well-known mahogany-colored Bacillus coli.

"It is Dr. Rife's belief that all micro-organisms fall into 1 of not more then 10 individual groups (Dr. Rosenow has stated that some of the viruses belong to the group of the streptococcus), and that any alteration of artificial media of slight metabolic variation in tissues will induce an organism of one group to change over into any other organism included in that same group, it being possible, incidentally, to carry such changes in media or tissues to the point where the organisms fail to respond to standard laboratory methods of diagnosis. These changes can be made to take place in as short a period of time as 48 hours. For instance, by altering the media - 4 parts per million per volume - the pure culture of mahogany-colored Bacillus coli becomes the turquoise-blue Bacillus typhosus. Viruses of primordial cells of organisms which would ordinarily require an 8-week incubation period to attain their filterable state, have been shown to produce disease within 3 days' time, proving Dr. Rife's contention that the incubation period of a micro-organism is really only a cycle of reversion.

He states:

"In reality, it is not the bacteria themselves that produce the disease, but we believe it is the chemical constituents of these micro-organisms enacting upon the unbalanced cell metabolism of the human body that in actuality produce the disease. We also believe if the metabolism of the human body is perfectly balanced or poised, it is susceptible to no disease."

"In other words, the human body itself is chemical in nature, being comprised of many chemical elements which provide the media upon which the wealth of bacteria normally present in the human system feed. These bacteria are able to reproduce. They, too, are composed of chemicals. Therefore, if the media upon which they feed, in this instance the chemicals or some portion of the chemicals

34

of the human body, become changed from the normal, it stands to reason that these same bacteria, or at least certain numbers of them, will also undergo a change chemically since they are now feeding upon media which are not normal to them, perhaps being supplied with too much or too little of what they need to maintain a normal existence. They change, passing usually through several stages of growth, emerging finally as some entirely new entity - as different morphologically as are the caterpillar and the butterfly (to use an illustration given us). The majority of the viruses have been definitely revealed as living organisms, foreign organisms it is true, but which once were normal inhabitants of the human body -living entities of a chemical nature of composition.

"Under the universal microscope disease organisms such as those of tuberculosis, cancer, sarcoma, streptococcus, typhoid, staphylococcus, leprosy, hoof and mouth disease, and others may be observed to succumb when exposed to certain lethal frequencies, coordinated with the particular frequencies peculiar to each individual organism, and directed upon them by rays covering a wide range of waves. By means of a camera attachment and a motion-picture camera not built into the instrument, many "still" micrographs as well as hundreds of feet of motion-picture film bear witness to the complete life cycles of numerous organisms. It should be emphasized, perhaps, that invariably the same organisms refract the same colors. when stained by means of the monochromatic beam of illumination of the universal microscope, regardless of the media upon which they re grown. The virus of the Bacillus typhosus is always a turquoise blue, the Bacillus coli always mahogany colored, the Mycobacterium leprae always a ruby shade, the filter-passing form of virus of tuberculosis always an emerald green, the virus of cancer always a purplish red, and so on. Thus, with the aid of this microscope, it is possible to reveal the typhoid organism, for instance, in the blood of a suspected typhoid patient 4 and 5 days before a Widal is positive. When it is desired to observe the flagella of the typhoid-organism, Hg salts are used as the medium to see at a magnification of 10,000 diameters.

"In the light of the amazing results obtainable with this universal microscope and its smaller brother scopes, there can be no doubt of the ability of these instruments to actually reveal any and all microorganisms according to their individual structure and chemical constituents.

"With the aid of its new eyes - the new microscopes, all of which are continually being improved - science has at last penetrated beyond the boundary of accepted theory and into the world of the viruses with the result that we can look forward to discovering new treatments and methods of combating the deadly organisms - for science dose not rest.

"To Dr. Karl K. Darrow, Dr. John A. Kolmer, Dr. William P. Lang, Dr. L. Marton, Dr. J. H. Renner, Dr. Royal R. Rife, Dr. Edward C. Rosenow, Dr. Arthur W. Yale, and Dr. V. K. Zworykin, we wish to express our appreciation for the help and information so kindly given us and to express our gratitude, also, for the interest shown in this effort of bringing to the attention of more of the medical profession the possibilities offered by the new microscopes."

In Rife's own words, here are other instruments he invented and used in his research: "The micromanipultor was used to dissect and operate on cells. The spectrometer was used to measure the angle of crystals; the frequency instruments were used to kill bacteria, virus, and fungi; and the microscopes of the prismatic virus were used to study living virus, bacteria, and fungi. A petrographical micropolariscope was used to analyze chemicals and color frequencies with polarized light, special rare gas glass contained atmospheres were used to provide ionized radiation to transmit energy to increase virulence and to devitalize all microorganisms as desired."

Rife concluded viruses were pathogenic by animal testing and from microscopic examination, which exposed the true identity of microorganisms to the trained observer, according to Rife's own comments. On one series of cancer tests, he inoculated the virus that he had isolated and filtered from an 'unulcerated' breast mass into an Albino rat. He then allowed the tumor to grow; then he surgically removed the tumor and again isolated and filtered the virus from a portion of the ground up tumor and inoculated the next rat and repeated this procedure 411 times to prove that this virus was causative agent of cancer. Tests on many other diseases such as those previously mentioned are too numerous to write about.

Rife concluded that a virus is released from bacteria just as a "chicken lays an egg." According to records, Rife found that bacillus coli, tuberculosis, typhoid and others were examples of some of the bacteria capable of releasing a form of virus.

A few of the physicians and scientists who were associated with Rife's experiments were: Milbank Johnson, M.D., Arthur I. Kendall, Ph.D., E.C. Rosenow, M.D., Coolidge of General Electric, O.C. Grunner, M.D., Henry Siner, Dr. Copp, M.D., Alvin G. Foord, M.D., Ernest Lynwood Walker, M.D., and Karl Meyer, M.D., of the Hooper Foundation of San Francisco, George Dock, M.D., Waylen Morrison, M.D., Dr. Fischer, M.D., Verne Thompson, Ben Cullen, Ray Lounsberry, M.D., James B. Couche, M.D., Charles F. Tully, D.D.S., Arthur Yale, M.D., R.T. Hamer, M.D., John Crane, Dave Sawyer, Don Tully, J. Heitger, M.D., Royal Lee, Ph.D., T.O. Burger, M.D., Alice Kendall and many others.

In order to complete his studies, he required completely different microscopes. He designed and built a prismatic virus microscope for virus study and research. He offered them to Bausch and Lomb, but they could not justify the cost of tooling to build these complex instruments, and the doctors could not afford to buy them either, because they were too expensive for the average laboratory to even consider, according to Rife.

Rife's extraordinary instruments showed the virus and allowed the researcher to study them alive and identify them as virus, and allow a diagnosis as to the disease of which they caused and were associated. He said the microscopes had to be of high enough power to enable the observer to see them and second they must be identified by a frequency of light, which coordinates with the chemical constituents of the virus or filterable form in question. "To my knowledge," Rife wrote, "there is only one instrument today which will even show these virus and that is the Rife prismatic virus microscopes which I built for this work. The electron microscope is a useless device for this study because the virus are killed instantly and you don't know what form you are seeing them in and generally appear as round balls of dried up chemical particles."

This author did not intend to bombard the reader with so many technical details, but how else can we show the seriousness and gravity of Rife's pursuit? By the way, the author of the scientific piece that was reprinted on these pages, Dr. Raymond Seidel, allegedly had at least one attempt made on his life, after numerous threats. It is not known whether that incident had anything to do with his article but he never wrote about Rife again.

4

Prince Edward Island, is the smallest of the Canadian provinces both in size and population. While it is densely populated, it is not overcrowded. The Province is also called 'PEI', or simply 'The Island'. They say that to be a 'true blue' Prince Edward Islander you must be born here. Otherwise, you're 'from away'. The capital city is Charlottetown. It is clean but congested. It has an ambience of its own, something special about it, like the French Quarter in New Orleans.

The 'Island way of life' is an often quoted and much discussed idea in Canada's small green province in the Gulf. For both Islanders and those 'from away' the quality of life on this island is the best. It is an ideal place to raise a family, to operate a business or to rejuvenate the mind, according to those who live here.

If lobster is the best food in the world, and many gourmands say it is, then PEI is a gourmand's heaven. Lobsters are abundant, relatively inexpensive and when served in a sparkling Acadian style restaurant, the most satisfying of meals. PEI is famous for "lobster suppers" and this also includes seafood chowder, mussels and soft clams. Tourists go there to see the Anne of Green Gables home and museum but they jam the better restaurants feasting on lobsters.

Lucy Maud Montgomery (1874-1942) made Anne the most famous character ever created in English literature. Mark Twain said that Anne is the greatest character ever portrayed in the English language. "Anne of Green Gables" was the first in a series of novels which cast a romantic glow over her native province and gained for her international fame as the creator of "one of the most loveable children in English fiction."

Anjanette desired to take her time on PEI, enjoying the sights and touring the island but that would have to wait until her business was concluded. She arrived in Charlottetown about 10:30am, after spending the night in Cape Tormentine in New Brunswick and then driving over the Confederation Bridge. She was disappointed to discover that the provincial government had made a storage house for bridge parts where her old home had stood.

In Charlottetown, she was instructed to go to Kent Street and there she would find the building where her attorneys are located. She had never met them. Actually, they were her attorneys only by default, as the attorneys were her Uncle Moreau's lawyers, the ones who handled the probate and settling of his estate. They had communicated by postal mail and email, only talking once on the telephone. She didn't know what to expect but was stunned to see the name on the building

41

was the same as on the letterhead: Speakman, Loebel, Silverstein and Meyer. The lawyer that contacted her was Herb Goldman.

Honestly, Anjanette did not know what the final settlement entailed. She knew about the rooming house but there was another property in the San Diego area she knew very little about, but it was vacant land, as far she knew, and the attorney had no appraisal done on its value. He did know the taxes were kept current and there were no mortgage or liens. She also expected 'a little money, not much, we don't know exactly' and tried to keep her expectations in check. She felt blessed and thankful that Uncle Moreau remembered her in this way.

The building was three stories tall and occupied entirely by the law firm. The receptionist said Anjanette was expected and she should take a seat. "Were you in an accident? Is that why you are seeing Mr. Goldman?" the receptionist wondered, noticing the crutches.

"I am here on a probate settlement-an inheritance." She ignored the reference to the accident. She dropped down deep into a thick, leather chair, and immediately regretted doing it. The chair was very low and low chairs were to be avoided, as they are extremely difficult to get out of without help. Anjanette did not like asking for help.

Nearly twenty minutes passed before the young receptionist advised Anjanette that she could now go into Goldman's office. While she was summoning her strength and courage to rise out of the chair without assistance, a young, dark man presented himself. "Hello, I am Herb Goldman," he said, smiling broadly. "I'm sorry to hold you out here Ms de la Houssaye, I did not know you had an accident." He reached down with both hands and helped Anjanette to her feet. "Was it very inconvenient for you to come?"

It was but she had no reason to tell him so. The airport at Vancouver was the first hurdle, but she surmounted it by requesting wheelchair assistance. Actually, she had the facility to walk all the way to the gate, even though it was the very last gate at the end of the concourse, but she had been delayed so long in security checks that she was tired, late and somewhat frustrated. Asking for the wheelchair meant she was giving in to her disability in her mind but she asked for it.

The next challenge was upon arrival at St. Johns, New Brunswick. Anjanette had reserved a specially equipped Chevrolet Suburban for her travels from there to PEI and back. She had a "guaranteed" reservation, with assurance the vehicle would be there awaiting her use upon arriving. It was not. A Suburban was there but it was not handicap equipped. "Take a seat and we will let you know when we locate the vehicle."

"I don't think so. I set this up three weeks ago. I have a guarantee in writing. I don't want to be unfair about this but I just cannot sit around this airport all afternoon. I have some driving to do to get where I am going," she said, obviously uncomfortable and irritated.

"All I can tell you is that we don't know yet where the vehicle is—when we find it—you can have it," the agent said, briskly walking away, leaving Anjanette there with her mouth open.

43

It was more than two hours before the vehicle showed up with no explanation offered as to why it was late or regret for the delay. But Goldman didn't need to know all of this.

———

Goldman's office was not as impressive as the building or outer surroundings. It was rather small, crowded with filing cabinets and a small conference table that used up too much of the space. In addition to the customary wall-mounted documents, he had several photos of himself skiing, swimming and snorkeling. Anjanette noticed different young women in each photo. "I never got the opportunity to ski," she said, nodding toward the photo while being seated with his assistance at the small conference table. He smiled warmly but said nothing. She offered no further explanation, although that was her intention.

He was young in appearance but he gave off an aura of confidence, as though this was something he had done many times, and that he knew what he was doing. A male secretary arrived with pots of coffee and tea. Anjanette accepted the tea. Goldman said nothing but the man poured a cup of very dark coffee. He left the room without a word said.

"Are you comfortable?"

"Yes, I'm fine. Thank you."

"May I call you Anjanette?"

"Anjie. My friends call me Anjie. I hope by the time I leave here that we are friends," she said, smiling.

"Absolutely, Anjie. Well, let's get on with it."

Spreading out two files with exact documents in each one, he explained the contents of the files and what had been done legally during the near-year it took to put matters to rest. "Don't worry," he winked, "we will get to the good part before the day is over!"

From the moment they met, Anjie liked Goldman. Yes, he is handsome but that was not all. He has an incredible personality and charisma. Goldman was most definitely very appealing to women but he did not seem arrogant or even aware of his power, she thought. As Goldman explained each document in the file and what it meant, he did it with a sense of seriousness with no hint of professor-student or parent-child, that one might be expecting from an attorney. He was businesslike but his voice was friendly.

Goldman was not from Canada but New York. He was graduated from Harvard University School of Law at 24. He considered teaching but then accepted a position with the law firm with the understanding that he would enter in the firm's 'quick recognition' program. At 28, he left New York for PEI, with the agreement that when he returned it would be as a junior partner.

Moreau was not his client and, in fact, he was unfamiliar with the file until a couple of weeks before this day with Anjie. A local attorney there at PEI was handling it for the firm but he left to enter medical school. Moreau was not the typical client of a prestigious

45

corporate law firm-he was actually a friend of a relative of a senior partner who had invested quite a lot of money with Moreau in the scientific device he was engineering in San Diego. The firm retained him because of these ties, otherwise there was no way that Goldman would have been handling a probate. He was a corporate attorney with special expertise in international joint ventures. Goldman actually sought out and acquired local assistance to help him wrap up the Moreau estate business for Anjie.

Ever since Anjie had met Horowitz, she also played the 'casting;' game of running characters through her mind and matching them up with actors. If Goldman made the story told in the TV movie, Anjie immediately thought of Benjamin Bratt.

"Anjie, I think we are at the good part now. Let me go over the main points for you: It is better than I led you to believe on the phone, but we still have a lot of unanswered questions. For one thing, we did not, because of the cost involved, officially appraise the property Moreau left you in California. We did have an economist-Realtor take a look at it, and her report stated an approximate value of $1.5 million. This number was accepted for the purposes of settling the estate."

"Incredible. I thought there was little money?"

"There is, in terms of actual cash or near cash, there is very little without a doubt. In fact, after all expenses of the court, attorney, accounting, and other fees, plus payment of all taxes, there is only $102.59 left. Moreau had very little by way of cash in savings or other accounts that we located. He did have some securities in what turned out to be worthless companies, with the exception of stock he purchased in the thirties that had multiplied through stock splits through the years. We liquidated that to pay all the expenses," he said dryly.

"There is the rooming house here in Charlottetown. It appraised for $750,000. There is an annual gross income of approximately $72,000. Moreau lived a very simple life in two rooms of the house; he has roomers that take care of things for reduced rent and other payments in kind. The house was inspected by licensed inspectors and their reports state the house is solid and pretty well cared for through the years." Quickly adding, "There are no mortgages or liens."

The idea of becoming an instant millionaire had never really entered her mind. From what she had been told, her expectations had been low. Within thirty minutes of entering the attorney's office, she is told in a very matter-of-fact way that she inherited a couple of million dollars of property. Her first thought was to view the property in San Diego. What she needed was money, and since that property was not producing income, she had wanted to sell it.

One thing for sure, she would not be returning to the newspaper. She was tired of journalism and of editing the 'petty' stories of small town government. The biggest issue she ever covered was whether the planning and zoning board should issue a permit to an American developer who wanted to build a five-story condo building. As it turned out, the board authorized the permit but the protest was so huge from the residents, they withdrew it six months later. The developer sued for $30 million and now the town is worried because they do not have $30 million, and they are self-insured. She definitely decided already she was not returning to that position.

"I am told Moreau's personal belongings are packed up for you, locked away in the basement at the rooming house. You may examine them whenever you wish, but there is nothing there of any significance in terms of value," Goldman said. "But I do have a new development here that worries me as we have closed the probate estate and now, the attorney who was handling this, sent a set of keys over to us by messenger yesterday. He wrote a note stating that one key is for the house and the other for a storage space rented by Moreau."

"Why is that troubling?"

"Only because if there is anything of value in the storage, we may have to reopen the file and notify the court," he said, shrugging his shoulders. "I should have gone to the storage center yesterday, but I worked on completing this file until late last night. The other attorney never bothered. All we can do is go see what is there, and what consequences result. Who knows? You may get very lucky and the place may be filled with valuables!"

"Could be, the way my luck is running today!" she said, smiling broadly, "I am very happy about all this news. It is very exhilarating and certainly unanticipated."

"Let's have lunch, then I will take you over to see the house-"

"-I prefer going in a straight line to the storage room, to get that done, and then I will know if I have room there to move items out of the house into storage. My preliminary thinking is that I will keep that house and even live in it—at least during the non-winter months. I plan to write a book!"

Goldman was under her scrutiny. She is fond of him but not just because of his looks, she appreciates his attitude and charisma. He is not so full of himself as he might be or as the politicians and business leaders of the town where she lived and worked. It had been a long time since she had any attraction to a man but she was feeling a special adrenaline flow.

"That is pretty much everything I have for you; it is all there in that file in front of you. All your legal documents." Looking a bit perplexed, he added, "I guess if you want to go to the storage barn, then we should head on out. We can lunch when we leave there."

———

The storage room shows no evidence of anything valuable or even useful. There were a few old radios, snow tires, winter weather gear, and assorted tools hung up on the wall. A broken chair, and a mattress that looked like it had never been unwrapped, and a small kitchen dining table with two chairs were stacked up in one corner. A shelf contained electrical sockets, light bulbs and wire. Another held plumbing and cleaning supplies. Goldman is drawn to a wall taken up with stacks of pipes, lenses, mirrors, couplings and thousands of other parts. "Look here, this looks like pieces of a telescope or something," he said, picking up one lens and then another for a closer look.

Anjie reacted immediately, but picking up an old worn leather briefcase in front of the stacked items. She unzipped it and found another wrapped package inside. Under the briefcase is a stack of schematic drawings and diagrams with engineering notations. "I wonder what these were for?" she said in a barely audible voice. "What do you think?"

Goldman acknowledged the long papers handed to him by Anjie but put them on the side while he scrutinize a giant lens more closely. "I have never seen so many lenses like this in my life. This must have been one hell of an instrument, whatever it was. How much do you know about this?"

"Very little. My mother told me about it and for years she and I received long, rambling letters from Moreau about an invention he was working on; but I was very young and then after the accident, frankly, I never paid much attention to it," she said.

"Do you have any documents or anything about this at home?"

"Probably. All the stuff he sent through the years is stored away. I really don't know what it all is."

"Get those newspapers down there, please, see what they say. They are wrapped in a way that they were intended to be preserved, but it is easier for you to grab them," Anjie said, nodding toward her crutches. The first one is the San Diego Tribune, May 6, 1938. The headline screamed out: "DREAD DISEASE GERMS DESTROYED BY RAYS, CLAIM OF S.D. SCIENTIST". A speed-reader, Goldman said the news story is about a scientist by the name of Royal Rife, a very powerful microscope and an instrument known as the Frequency Generator. Goldman continued reading the other papers. "Look at this story, a meeting to discuss "The End of All Diseases"! Anjie remembered the package left in the briefcase. Using her teeth for help, she unwrapped the dusty package.

"It's a diary, the diary of Henry Moreau, my uncle", Anjie exclaimed. Goldman dropped the papers gently to the floor to see what Anjie had. "Here's a letter inside addressed to Uncle Moreau signed by Royal Rife, the scientist mentioned in those newspaper stories." She commenced to read it aloud:

"We completed the first instrument in 1920 at a cost of about $35,000, you will remember I told you this was possible only because of Maime and Ah Quin, her father. This version of the microscope, you will remember, contained exactly 5,682 parts and it weighed nearly 200 pounds. By 1935, after you went back to Canada, we had simplified the machine by reducing the number of parts. I am sending these parts to you for safekeeping. The pharma-medical cartel is doing everything in its power to prevent the cancer cure from being tested by the independent labs. You will be glad to know that we were successful with the Frequency Generator. I actually discovered the lethal frequency for a number of different disease organisms, which blew them up, killing them. For example, Typhoid, E-coli, TB,

51

Pneumonia, and many others. If anything happens to me and it will, you are the only person I trust who is still living who has the ability to rebuild the microscope and frequency generator. Whether the diseases get cured or not may end up depending upon your success." Then both together, they read the last sentence of the letter aloud: "All the cancer patients tested at my lab under the auspices of USC are cured."

Speechless, Anjie and Goldman stand virtually motionless, reading and rereading the letter. Anjie begins thumbing through the diary. "Here, look, it refers to a Dr. Cyrus Cleveland who was an associate of Moreau and Rife." According to the diary, they both lived in a retirement home together. "This means there is a living link to what Moreau and Rife did. This guy, if he is still alive, he can tell us more about all of this."

"But why? What can we do about it?"

"IF we have parts and the drawings, and if we knew what we were doing, wouldn't it be possible to rebuild the microscope and frequency generator? What if it is true that they discovered a way of curing diseases, including cancer?"

"Without drugs? I think we are both worldly enough to know that any cure not involving drugs leaves out the hospitals, the doctors, the research, the non-profit fund raising, insurance companies and, of course, the pharmaceutical companies that develop and make the drugs. What?"

"-Wait, you just answered our own questions. How could such an invention be allowed? There is probably too much money at stake involving too many people."

"We don't have the expertise to deal with this. I don't know about you, but I can look at those parts and schematics all day, and not ever know what it is all about. We do not have any chance to delve into this or to even think about it-"

"-Not so. We must think about it. What if someone had a cure for paralysis and it was concealed and I suffered all my life unnecessarily? Think of the millions of people all over the world who die from cancer and other diseases, who probably can't even afford the drugs or treatments prescribed. This is destiny; my destiny at least-I cannot limp away from here like nothing has happened. We have a Christian obligation to pursue it!," she said adamantly.

Smiling and looking somewhat sheepish, Goldman said, "Oh, well, I guess that explains it for you but what about me?"

"OK, so I guess that means you are not Christian! Let me rephrase what I said: We have a Judeo-Christian obligation to see where all of this takes us. And thanks to Uncle Moreau, I have the time and money to do it. If you cannot help, I will understand."

"If Rife was in danger, what do you think could happen to us?," he asked.

"We can't think about that, at least we can't think about it now."

5

Rancho Santa Fe is definitely at the high-end of real estate values in San Diego. The average price of a home is well over $2-million and trending up at an incredible average of about 7 percent a year. Actually Rancho Santa Fe is a conglomeration of communities and country clubs and is unincorporated. Included within Rancho Santa Fe are Fairbanks Ranch and the country club communities of Del Mar, Morgan Run and another in the planning stage. The area is wealthy and prestigious. Worth Magazine once rated Rancho Santa Fe as the sixth richest community in the country. Established about 70 years ago, the housing is a mix of old, fairly old and new, with the newer homes in Fairbanks Ranch and Del Mar. The property inherited by Anjie is a vacant but lot located in the oldest section, a property intended for commercial exploitation at a corner and on busy streets.

Anjie is told by a Realtor that she recommends listing the property for sale at $2-million. "You will get close to it," the Realtor promised. Anjie thought about listing it right then but she did not like the

Realtor who seemed overly confident and cocky, especially for a woman in her early twenties. The woman, calling herself "Sudsy" Lanahan, dressed and looked more like a dancer in a men's club then she did a Realtor. She wore a too short and tight skirt with a halter, just barely covered up by a light blue blazer. She spoke fast and didn't seem to listen to anything Anjie said.

"You are a Canadian and we have a lot of what we call 'snow birds' down here in the winter. Most of them come down to enjoy the weather and activities but since you are handicapped, I don't know, I imagine it doesn't much matter where you live," she blurted out en route to the property. "I mean, you know, you don't ski or take long walks on the ocean, I guess."

Anjie remained silent, but grinding her teeth so she would not open her mouth.

The Mercedes they were riding in was small and uncomfortable for Anjie and more than once "Sudsy" was asked to slow it down by Anjie who did not like being so low to the ground and traveling fast in traffic. The driver's response was to mutter something.

"The concierge at the Del Coronado is a very good friend of mine. I stop there quite often for drinks; I live in Coronado. I am glad he called me as I am quite familiar with the area where your property is located," pausing, "you do have title to it, right? Otherwise we are wasting our time."

Anjie did not reply but she nodded yes. "I am sure if it is a vacant lot, it is one of the few vacant lots out there. What really happens in the older sections of Rancho Santa Fe is that people buy a property out there with an old house on it and tear it down. Can you imagine tearing down a million dollar house? It happens here all the time. I don't guess you ever heard of anything like that in Canada?"

Anjie nearly told her about the soaring values of properties in British Columbia, especially near Vancouver, but she decided against it. She would see the property and then decide what do with it. She was in no hurry.

She promised to call Herb Goldman at PEI after seeing it. She could hardly wait to make that call.

––––––––

"L.M. Montgomery, the author of Anne of Green Gables, was born on the north shore of Prince Edward Island and raised in Cavendish where she lived until she married at the age of 36," the museum guide said. "Anne of Green Gables has been translated into 15 different languages and put on film. The land, the sea and the people on PEI inspired the original story. Anne is responsible for drawing more than 350,000 visitors annual from all around the world to PEI, nearly all of them wanting to see the Green Gables House."

"I am pleased you are taking the time to see this," Goldman said, "as it is the main attraction on PEI. Frankly, there is not much to do here, if you don't like lobsters and Anne of Green Gables," he smiled.

"Besides, you need to get your mind off that stuff in the storage locker."

"That will not happen. I can't think about anything else and I wonder how you can!"

"Because I am young and want to live, besides I have other things to do and think about-"

"-Like I don't? I just inherited a fortune and you think I have nothing else to think about?"

"No, I don't mean that. What I mean is that even if I wanted to help you, I don't know where to start. I am not an engineer, and you are thinking about a difficult, long- term project that could become quite costly. Frankly, we just don't have enough to go on-"

"-You don't but I do. I have seen enough to know that I want to read every word of that dairy and look over those schematics and plans. Maybe it is a pipe dream, one that Moreau spent his life working on with Rife; but I owe it to him to try to find out if there is any truth to it."

"What are you going to do?"

"Go to San Diego. I have two reasons to go now, the first is to see the property to decide what to do with it, and the other is to try to locate Dr. Cleveland, if he is still alive."

"I can understand that but until you leave, why don't I just take as much time as possible to show you around?"

"Only if you promise to go through that diary with me," she said.

———

Using a spare office at the law firm, Anjie spread out the newspapers from the storage room, read one and then handed it to Goldman. The date was November 22, 1931, and the paper was the Los Angeles Times. "Scientific discoveries of the greatest magnitude, including a discussion of the world's most powerful microscope recently perfected after 14 years of effort by Dr. Royal Rife of San Diego, were described Friday evening to members of the medical profession, bacteriologists and pathologists, at a dinner given by Dr. Milbank Johnson in honor of Dr. Rife and Dr. A. I. Kendall.

"Through the use of Dr. Rife's powerful microscope, said to have a visual power of magnification to 17,000 times, compared with 2,000 times which the ordinary microscope is capable, Dr. Kendall said he could see the typhoid bacilli in the filterable or formerly invisible stage. It is probably the first time the minute filterable virus organisms have been seen."

"I'm not a doctor or engineer but seeing this type of reporting in the Los Angeles Times convinces me that there probably is something to all of this about Rife and the cures. I am more concerned about it now then I was before. I can see where this hcadcd right into conflict with the pharmaceutical-medical establishment," Goldman said.

Reading from the diary, Anjie responded: "Dr. Royal Lee of the Lee Foundation for Nutritional Research spent a lot of time with me at my lab. He later criticized the AMA and Dr. Fisbein for not publishing stories about my inventions and research. Lee found out for himself what I had been telling him: Censorship is strictly applied when research is directed away from drugs."

"Hear this," she ordered, "this is where he summarizes in a sentence all that he did: "In reality, it is not the bacteria themselves that produce the disease, but the chemical constituents of the micro-organisms enacting upon the unbalanced cell metabolism of the human body that in actuality produces the disease of cancer. We also believe that if the metabolism of the human body is perfectly balanced or poised it is susceptible to no disease."

"I just don't know what we can do. Even if there is something to all of this-"

"-I think we need to inventory the parts we have of the instruments from storage as best we can, gather up the engineering drawings and write ups that we found, and take all of it with the diary to an engineer that we can trust, and then take it one step at a time," she said. "Whatever the consequences."

Sliding over to where Anjie was sitting at a desk, he looked at her earnestly, quietly, for a period of time. She did not interrupt the silence. Eventually, he started nodding his head sideways. "You realize this is a fantasy. It may even have been a hoax. These people, we don't know them, they may have used all of this to scam money from investors. Maybe the people pursuing them were not members of the pharmaceutical-medical industry but those who had their wallets lifted."

"Perhaps. I can't even vouch for my uncle, much less Royal Rife. Maybe this is all hocus-pocus. But if we leave it, can you honestly say that you will never look back and regret that you didn't try to find out?"

"Anjie, I can't say that. God-knows I may end up regretting inaction. There is always the possibility, no matter how remote, that there is some truth to all of this. But I don't think the way to proceed is to gather this stuff up and find an engineer-"

"-Well, how?"

"Let's leave it in safe storage where it has been for all these years. The first thing we should do is find anyone we can whose name is mentioned that is still alive-"

"-Yea, Dr. Cleveland in San Diego, for example."

"Exactly."

"Let's see if we find out anything worth pursuing. If we do, then we go to the next step, that being reassembling or trying to reassemble the instruments. If not, we forget about it," he said firmly.

Closing the diary and again neatly stacking the newspapers, Anjie nodded agreement.

"I understand you can't get up and go to San Diego. I want to view the property. I will look up Dr. Cleveland and if that develops positively, I will call you. It will be up to you as to what you do next," she said.

"Fair enough. Look, I am not sure I should ask, but this disability you have-"

"Swimming accident when I was twelve years old. I dived into the shallow end of a pond that was only three feet deep; a spinal chord injury was the outcome. But I am lucky-consider what happened to Christopher Reeves! I regained a lot of my skills through rigorous rehabilitation over the years. I'm OK, really..." This was a sort of speech that Anjie used frequently when the subject finally arises.

"I just wanted to know how serious it is. You seem fine and you do not let it keep you from doing what needs done," Goldman said, somewhat patronizingly.

"I can't let it get me down. I am past all of that. I am over it and now I accept it. I live with it and make the most of it. Don't worry; I can travel to San Diego or anywhere without any assistance. I rarely encounter difficulties," she said, testily.

"Wow!" Goldman exclaimed, smiling broadly. "I expected that from you!"

"Wow! Right!" she said, smiling. "Now you know!"

———

"San Diego has so many distractions, I admit that I have not spent the time on the investigation of the Rife machine as I thought I would," Anjie admitted. "I guess now that I am a member of the wealthy class, I am getting lazy," she said, frowning. "I am glad you are here."

Herb Goldman arrived in San Diego only three days after Anjie. He had told her it would take him a week or more to clear his business obligations, but when he advised a senior partner in the firm what he was interested in doing, he was urged to get started.

"I hope you don't mind that I am staying in Coronado. I couldn't resist the temptation of staying at the Del Coronado where all the movies have been made, although I must admit that at $600 a day, I cannot stay much longer-"

"-Anjie, have you forgotten, you are rich now?"

"Rich? But without money. I am using my VISA card that is dangerously close to its limit. I am projecting that I can stay here another three or four days before my credit card is topped out," she groaned. "Any ideas?"

"Of course, I will get the firm to advance you $50,000 or so. We can place a lien on your property in PEI or a simple first mortgage on your property in California. Or I may even get them to do it without all that paper work, just by you signing a note."

Herb was dressed casually, the first time Anjie had seem him without a tie. He looked bigger, more athletic than he did in PEI and in excellent physical condition. He wore a dark blue blazer with the insignia of Harvard University but he avoided a preppy look. They were in a limo hired by the firm to pick up Anjie and then Herb at the airport, en route to Coronado. It was early in the afternoon. Anjie wanted to compliment Herb on his appearance but she was not certain how to do it. The opportunity presented itself.

"You look fabulous, Anjie. I can certainly see how all that rehabbing toned up your body. You should be doing TV commercials," he said, shyly.

"Thank you. You are also pretty," she said, laughing.

The limo pulled up in the front of the hotel. The driver asked if there were any services that were desired. "Yes, please, stand by. We would like to go out to Rancho Santa Fe after Herb gets checked in. You can wait out here or in the lobby, we will only be a few minutes," she said.

Anjie called Sudsy to meet them at Rancho Santa Fe but not at the property, as Anjie did not know how to find it. They agreed to meet for lunch at a chic Italian restaurant near where they were going. As a well-known landmark, Sudsy said, the driver will have no trouble finding it. Almost immediately upon arriving at the restaurant, Anjie realized she had made a blunder in inviting the Realtor.

Wearing a form fitting tight white dress that exposed as much as possible of her long legs and highlighted her large black designer sunglasses, the Realtor looked liked a movie star. From the very second Herb and Sudsy met, Anjie felt electricity go through the air. Herb was enthralled by her, even moved speechless for a few minutes. She was openly flirting with him. This was not the luncheon that Anjie had in mind.

While Anjie did all she could to stay on topic, Herb listened intently to Sudsy who told of local nightspots that were great for dancing and long evenings out. She suggested meeting Herb and

Anjie later that night after dinner. "But I guess you are not interested in dancing, are you?"

The words hung in Anjie's ears and pounded her eardrums relentlessly. Before she could react, Herb did. "Anjie is a better athlete than the two of us together, but she does her exercising in the pool. But if she would like to go, well-"

"-No, but I don't want you to miss the opportunity. Have fun. We have tomorrow to do what we came here to do," Anjie said, trying her best to sound very disinterested in the proposed date later that night.

"Fine," Sudsy said, cheerily. "It is settled. You wont need that limo-I live in Coronado-I will pick you up about 9:00pm. Now let's discuss the property."

They did. Although it was clearly not her desire or intention, Anjie decided to list the property with Sudsy for sale. Herb did not interfere in any way or even make a suggestion as to listing it, but he was obviously delighted to get it done with Sudsy. Anjie sat quietly, smiling but not liking the idea of Sudsy with Herb.

Sudsy produced the listing form from her briefcase and proceeded to fill it in. "Anjie, all I need from you right now is your signature-"

"-I can get you the legal documents showing ownership, etc. I will have them sent down via Fed Ex tomorrow," Herb interrupted.

It was done. Anjie's property in San Diego was listed for $1.9 million. Sudsy predicted Anjie could hold out for that price. Herb smiled.

Later that night, alone in the hotel suite, Anjie could not even remember what they ate for lunch. All she could remember was Herb ogling Sudsy's silicone boobs bouncing around all during the meal. For the first time in her life, Anjie was jealous of another woman.

6

Anjie and Herb spent only a little time together at the rooming house she inherited. After meeting the residents and the 'acting manager', Anjie toured the building with Herb. Her main interest was in finding the personal belongings of Moreau that were packed up in the basement and going through them. She acknowledge to Herb that she was now practically single-mindedly thinking of the Rife invention, and the significance of the story.

Anjie hurriedly decides that she does not want to live in that house. It is too big, too old, too warm in the summer and probably too cold in the winter. It was dull, colorless and musty. It wasn't unexpected, but Anjie had hoped for a nice suite where she could live comfortably; there wasn't any; the house had been cut into one and two room sections for renting.

The 'estate' had appointed one of the roomers as the 'acting manager' in exchange for rent cut in half. The man, about 75, was tall, dirty and grossly overweight. His first words to Anjie upon meeting her were: "If you want me to stay in this job, you have to give me more money by eliminating my rent." She smiled but said nothing.

A young woman in her early twenties arrived shortly after Anjie. She said she was a teacher from New Orleans who was up there to study French. "Shouldn't you be over in New Brunswick or even Quebec? Less than one percent of the population in PEI speaks and writes French.

"Maybe, but I like it here. It is easier to meet people," she said, matter-of-factly. "You know, I don't like all work with no play!" She started to walk away, but then turned to Anjie: "Are you staying here tonight? Maybe we can have a glass of wine or something together," she said, smiling.

At that moment Anjie made her decision. "No, actually, I am staying somewhere else. But I will be in and out over the next few days," she said. The very next day, she and Herb hired a real estate management company.

———

It was dark in San Diego and from her balcony at the Del Coronado, Anjie watched the lights twinkle from ships at sea. Directly beneath her balcony was an outdoor restaurant that was packed with visitors drinking, eating and dancing to the music of a Latin quartet. She was lonely but hated admitting it. She resisted as much as possible thinking about Herb and Sudsy, out that evening dancing.

Herb stopped by the suite to invite Anjie to dinner or drinks, before he left for the evening, but she declined. She was ordering room service. He appeared disappointed when he left. Anjie later wished she had said yes. After suffering through years of rehabilitation and depression, she knew how to recognize the onset of trouble and that night, on that cool resort balcony, she was beginning to sense trouble. Trouble to Anjie meant negative thoughts. Everything she accomplished since her accident was attributable to positive thinking. She knew it was time to get back to basics. Silently at first she reiterated her little personal prayer. Then aloud, she said: "God, I know I am responsible for the experiences and events in my life. When I see them for what they are, I can control them. My inner voice, all too often, is pretty negative. I'm in control, and I can do it. I no longer hear that voice that says 'I can't.'"

After repeating several times, she felt better. The only thing missing from her regimen was a full body message.

She turned her attention and energy to Rife's invention, and what she could do while in San Diego. She decided to find Dr. Cleveland. That was priority one, but she also came to another decision: She is thinking about Herb with Sudsy. She wasn't going to give up so quickly.

"Having spent every dime I earned in my research for the benefit of mankind, I have ended up a pauper, but I achieved the impossible and would do it again," Rife wrote. The words stick to Anjie like glue. Rife said that the medical association "brainwashed and intimidated" his colleagues as well as "feloniously censored" the publication of his work. Rife was certain beyond a doubt that the national and federal health associations "declared war" on his inventions.

"We cannot just skip through this diary, ignoring what is written. Even if only half of it is true, it is a historical travesty that must be verified and, if possible, corrected," Anjie said, working at her desk in the suite. "Do you agree?"

"Yes, you know I do. I just don't know how far we can go. All of this supposedly happened a long time ago. The trail may be too cold," Herb shrugged.

"I know but listen to what he writes: 'Independent scientists and physicians are on record as having success with my Rife Frequency Generator in curing cancer and other diseases, as well as skin ailments. I have the affidavits on file. The Government and the medical associations know this but they will not take it into consideration.'"

Rife also noted that Dr. Cleveland, a research associate, is a qualified physician who has proof of the effectiveness of the Rife Frequency Generator. "Cleveland worked directly with Harry F.

69

Simon of the George William Hooper Foundation, one of the earliest research organizations formed to cure cancer, and they hailed the device for its effectiveness against typhoid organisms."

"The problem, Herb said, "is that when the State Department of Health said that the claims they reviewed were rejected by them because the testimonials were 'unverified', that may be correct; and that there was a lack of 'clinical evidence', it could be that they are telling the truth; it may be Rife who is misstating the facts."

"Exactly. I am not saying that this diary is a Bible, or that it is a prayer book. But I think we owe it to ourselves and dare I say it, humanity?, to find out what we can, since it seems like it is left up to us," Anjie said. "I think we have an obligation that goes beyond our own self-interests," she said, convincingly. "I am not even swayed by the words my uncle wrote here, where he swears that he and Rife became 'men of faith', and they grew to love Jesus in their later years."

"Anjie, I did some research after you left PEI. I discovered something interesting that lends credibility to the idea that a conspiracy did exist to prevent a cancer cure that does not involve drug therapy," Herb said, retrieving a file folder from his briefcase. "Read this."

The document was a reprint of an article published March 2, 1992 in Barron's. In the article David Kessler, who was once the head of the Food and Drug Administration, admitted that payoffs might be taken. He is quoted as saying: "Everything is tainted. Almost every doctor in academia has something going on the side, and I don't know what it is. I don't have the authority to find out. I don't know what they are getting legally as far as financial return, stock, money, whatever, I certainly don't know what they are getting under the table."

"Cancer is big business. It represents up to $75 billion annually in terms of hard cash. I have a friend at a university in Boston; who admitted to me that if a therapy existed for cancer that did not involve drugs, and it replaced Chemotherapy, that the number of bankruptcies that erupted in the medical profession, including medical schools where research is done, would be unbelievable and a severe blow to Wall Street, so severe it would take years to recover," Herb said.

"I think all we are doing now is sitting around this $600 a day suite convincing ourselves, and it is sounding more and more like we are both convinced. If this is the case, then I suggest we take off after Dr. Cleveland, but we must keep this absolutely confidential as any outside disclosures are potentially harmful to our health," she said.

"I agree but I must admit I have discussed this in non-specific terms with certain persons-" "-Like what persons?"

"Seniors at my law firm. One of the partners—Mr. Loebel - had a father, who invested money with Rife, and they believed in Rife, but they don't know why the thing failed. I also mentioned it to a few academics up in Boston," he said.

"You mean you discussed this with physicians in medical research at Harvard?"

"I didn't say Harvard. Just friends: I don't see that it matters, in as much as what can they do about it? They don't know what information we have."

"Right but they talk, and others talk and before long-"

"-You are assuming now that there is a pharmaceutical-medical conspiracy against Rife and his inventions—even today. Isn't that premature?"

"Premature. At PEI, you were also concerned about security, weren't you? After what you just showed me, I would think you are even more worried," she said, obviously irritated.

"OK, let's start over. I probably did discuss this with too many people in Boston, Canada, New York and even here-"

"-Here? Well, yes, I told Sudsy why I was here. She was wondering if we had some sort of romantic thing going on and if so, why was I out with her, but I set her right and told her that I was here on business. I was the attorney who handled your uncle's estate, and that we came here about the Rife inventions-"

Pulling herself up as quickly as possible from the desk, Anjie exploded. "I can't believe it. You told Sudsy? I cannot imagine that you would share this type of confidential and personal information with that air head-"

"-Air head? Is that what you have against her?"

"I don't owe you an explanation, I am just too upset to think about it. Why don't we take a break from each other for a while? Maybe you should go back to PEI and let me handle my own business here."

"Go back? No way. I agree we need a break. Why don't we order up some coffee or something and let it go at that?"

"No, I think I need some privacy. The thought of you sitting around a disco with that slutty looking b- talking about my uncle, Rife and me, is a bit more than I can stand."

Herb put an arm around Anjie. Gently, he whispered into her ear. "If I knew you better, I would suspect that you may have more than one reason to dislike Sudsy. Are you jealous that I spent the evening with her?"

"Evening? Wasn't it more like night?"

"What?"

"You heard me. I called you at 7 o'clock this morning in your room; there was no answer-"

"Oh, OK, well, I am beginning to see now what this may be about. I was out all night-"

"-Forget it. I don't want to hear about it; it is none of my business. Let's get together in an hour or so. In the meantime, I will get the address of the nursing home where this Dr. Cleveland is, and we can go there and get this over with," she said.

"One hour," he said, smiling smugly.

7

Anjie and Herb regard each other with uncertainty as he starts toward her in the lobby of the Del Coronado. In a way, they are meeting for the first time. After all that has happened since they first met in Charlottetown, neither can be certain of the others' feelings. It is a time of uneasiness and caution, eventually giving way to what has always been apparent: the fact that they do like each other more than somewhat. A moment of silence and then they move closer.

Angie agonized over this moment for the past hour. She is embarrassed by Herb staying out all night with Sudsy. Anjie is not sure she wants to make peace with him. Angie's heart is pounding as though it is about to explode. The tension is eased by the sound of the limo driver's voice: "Here I am. Are you folks ready to go?"

Anjie and Herb eased their way into the limo without a word. They sat silently for several minutes. "Where are we going?," asked the driver. Anjie hears the hint of an accent. She passes the address to Herb who slips it through the open partition. "No problem. I know where this is. It will take about an hour this time of the evening," he said, raising the glass partition between he and his passengers.

"This is the busiest time of the day. But I guess we should go see Dr. Cleveland before he dies!," Herb says, somewhat sarcastically.

Anjie says nothing for a few minutes. "Are you in a hurry?," she asked. "Do you have a date tonight?"

Laughing, Herb responded by nodding his head yes. When he drew the negative nods from Anjie he anticipated, he smiled and touched her hand. "With you. I heard of a great place for dinner tonight."

"I'm not your type. If we go to dinner, you will be expecting to spend the night with me in my bed," she said, slightly smiling.

"Oh, you have me figured out alright. That would be great. Are you certain we cannot plan on it?"

"Positively!"

"Well, sometimes I make exceptions, and actually go out with someone just because I like them. Suppose we go just for that reason?"

"We can but we won't. Besides, even if you do like me, that doesn't mean I like you. In fact, I am thinking right now that I probably don't like you," she said. "I bet that is a big blow to your rather inflated ego, especially after all the crap you were fed last night by sweet thing."

"Not that it is any of your business, but I was pretty bored with sweet thing after the first hour or so. Her range of interests is very small. She insisted we drive up the coast to a place that stays open all night, and that is what we did. That was all there was to it," he said, nodding his head affirmatively.

"You're right, it is none of my business. I'm sorry for the attitude. Let's forget about this and get down to business."

Herb smiled. He agreed.

———

"With the frequency instrument treatment, no tissue is destroyed, no pain is felt, no noise is audible, and no sensation is noticed. A tube lights up and 3 minutes later the treatment is completed. The virus or bacteria is destroyed and the body then recovers itself naturally from the toxic effect of the virus or bacteria. Several diseases may be treated simultaneously."

"This statement appears in a diary left by my Uncle Moreau. It was written, according to him, by Royal Rife," Anjie said, reading the statement and handing Dr. Cleveland a copy. The old man just smiled, saying nothing.

Growing impatient, Herb asked, "Well, what do you say? Is this correct?"

There wasn't any doubt that Dr. Cleveland heard them or that he understood. Although advanced in years, he had full control over his

76

body and mind, from what Herb and Anjie were told by nursing home attendants. They were warned, however: "If he gets angry with you, take off and get out of his way. He will throw whatever is near him!"

"I don't get it," he said, finally. "What is this all about?"

"We advised you that we are researching to write a book about Royal Rife. You are a living person who worked with and knew him. We are interviewing you for this reason," Anjie said, hoping the old man understood the reasons.

"I may be old and ugly," he said, looking into the mirror in his room, "but I'm not crazy. I've already had several phone calls that you people were making inquiries up in Boston and New York about Rife and his work, and what happened. I knew it was impossible to keep his work quiet forever."

Anjie flushed red and nodded her head negatively at Herb. She was right; there was no way that this secret would be kept once it went past the two of them. Anjie and Herb leveled with Dr. Cleveland. They told him they were there because they had what they were thinking (and hoping?) were the parts or pieces, that made up the microscope and the Frequency Generator. They wanted to know two things: 1). Is it true they cured diseases? and 2). Can the instruments be rebuilt?

Cleveland's room was surprisingly more than a room. It was like a suite in a hotel with a nice sitting area with a sofa and chairs, and a desk with a laptop computer on top. Cleveland's suite was on the third floor, but with a balcony, overlooking a beautifully maintained green space with a view of the Santa Monica Mountains in the distance. It was bright and colorful. Cleveland saw the curiosity his visitors had about the place. "This is not just a nursing home. There is a portion of the complex devoted to 24//7 care, but I live in the assisted care section. In other words, I have someone to see that I take my meds on time, and to aggravate me about when and what to eat, but otherwise I am on my own."

"This must cost a lot of money," Herb blurted out, wishing he hadn't. Anjie stared at him in disbelief. "It did. It is one of those deals where you pay upfront an agreed amount, and then you can stay as long as you live, with absolutely no living expenses except for incidentals. At the rate I am going, they will go broke with me," he chuckled.

"What about the questions we asked, Dr. Cleveland?," Anjie asked.

"I am remiss if I do not caution you that you are playing in a very dangerous game. For many years now, the enemies of Rife and his inventions assumed that the instruments were lost, and all the documentation having to do with their construction was destroyed, lost or stolen. As soon as these people find out this is not true, you two are in danger," he said slowly, seriously. "In fact, if I knew you had the stuff, even before you left Prince Edward Island, you can believe others also know, and this is not good for any of us. As for me, I am an old man who lived my life. You two are a young couple that have many years ahead-"

"-I am not afraid. For one thing, I had a totally debilitating accident when I was twelve years old. I was told I would never walk again. I overcame that fear, and now I am not afraid of anything," Anjie said.

Herb, looking at Anjie with admiration, said "I guess I am also a fighter. I had to overcome poor parenting, having a mother who had less than eight years of schooling, and a father who was in jail as much as he was home. I won scholarships to prep schools and Yale University, and then took a law degree from Harvard without paying a penny. I don't think I 'm afraid of anything, either."

Anjie is astonished by Herb's disclosures. She had speculated he was from a wealthy East Coast family, and the second or third generation at Harvard Law. She said nothing, choosing to let it pass, as he did her remarks about her childhood accident.

"You kids are the type of children I wish I had had. If I had gotten married to a woman instead of Rife and his projects, well, I probably would have had a couple of kids," Cleveland said.

"About the instruments: The answers to your questions are yes and yes. All things are possible in science, but I can tell you that it is highly unlikely—virtually impossible—that you can rebuild the instruments. But, yes, sadly—very sadly—it is true that Rife cured cancer and other diseases as well."

Anjie and Herb each smiled and nodded. "Then it was all true," Anjie said, adding, "but some type of conspiracy prevented the device from being tested nationally?"

"Honey, I am too old and don't have enough time to tell you that whole story. But if you have a diary, then, you probably know what happened. Simply stated, when it became obvious from the testing we were curing animals, and the 20 physicians using our instruments were curing patients, the theory appeared legitimate, well—from that moment on, the Establishment of Medicine and Pharmaceuticals—the whole medical industry—ganged up on us and shut us down."

Cleveland becomes animated. He leaps up and paces the floor, his head down the entire time he is talking. "I can tell you this first hand. Dr. Morris Fishbein was the head of the AMA at the time, and the editor of the Journal. Nothing got past him. From 1924 until 1949, Fish *was* the AMA. Remember, during this time there was no drug-testing agency like the FDA. Fish decided what doctors heard about drugs, and even more importantly, he decided on what drugs. He was the most powerful man in medicine."

"Are you saying that one man prevented Rife's inventions from being applied to curing diseases or even verifying your testing," Anjie asked, incredulously.

"I'm saying that without Fishbein's support, and without articles in the Journal, there wasn't any way we could get any credibility or legitimacy. I can't tell you why it happened, I heard different stories of why Fish did what he did, but I cannot testify to either of them-"

"What do you know?" Anjie interrupted. "Tell us, please."

"It is no secret that Fish had a lot of money. He liked money. An attorney came to us one day—your uncle was there. He tried to buy stock in our marketing company. He hinted he knew all the right people including Fishbein. We were all convinced Fish sent him, but we didn't know and we had no way of finding out. When we asked him, he didn't actually deny it; he only said that he could not tell us who sent him. Maybe we were paranoid. I don't know. I do know that Fish saw himself as the most vigorous crusader against quackery of his time. Quackery was whatever he said it was. He saw himself as the creator of what we know as the pharmaceutical-medical complex. In the public's perception, he is probably a great man," Cleveland said, finally raising his head and walking over to Anjie. "He was a dictator who got what he wanted."

"I believe Fishbein may have wanted the stock in the company but for reasons other than what you think. He may have wanted to get a closer look at the invention, or something like that," Herb said. "In other words, it may have been a positive thing. You apparently saw it as a 'bribe' type thing-".

"-I wouldn't say that," Cleveland responded, "Rife was more suspicious than Moreau or myself but he had reason to be, since we were experiencing losses in our lab, and life was generally pretty frustrating for us."

Chuckling, Cleveland took Herb and Anjie both by the arms. "You have to understand those decades and you cannot possibly, because of your ages. Hell, soon after Fish took over the AMA, he changed the name of one of the most important functions of the new organization. He changed the name of the Propaganda Department to the Bureau of Investigation. What does that tell you?"

Anjie and Herb were speechless. The old man dropped down into a chair at the desk and swiveled over to where they were standing. "From what I hear and read, modern day AIDS research is based on many of the same principles we created in our research. I have no doubt that Rife demonstrated time after time—and so did other competent researchers and physicians—that his theories, when tested properly, resulted in curing cancer and other diseases...but now I think it is time you young people go on with your lives. My advice is to forget all of this."

"Forget? How can we?," Anjie asked. "I am very very sorry that our carelessness caused the news to get out that we have these documents and instrument parts at Prince Edward Island. It was a mistake. This has caused you to be cautious about what you tell us, and I understand why. But all of this leads us to one final question: IF we do have all the documents and parts we need to put it all together, will you help us?"

"Lady, I am an old man; there are days when I am awake for only about six hours! Maybe that is an exaggeration but not by much. You cannot rely on me. There is a woman; she must be in her fifties now; she was once in love with Rife, after his beloved Maime died. She was an optical engineer who had met Rife in Germany when he was over working for Zeuss and doing some lecturing at Heidelberg

University. She was a student when he was already an old man. If you can find her, she may help-"

"What is her name or do you know where she is?" Herb asked.

"Her name is Gertrude Milhaus. She was an extremely brilliant engineer, and it was many of her ideas that Rife accepted. She knew those instruments from beginning to end. She was living right out here in Southern California, back then she lived in Pt. Loma where Rife lived, but she is surely gone from there by now. She had several advantages, all to Rife's liking: She was independently wealthy, having inherited a fortune from someone in Germany; she was very beautiful; and she was about 25 or more years younger than Royal!"

"What happened to her?" Anjie asked.

"When Rife started having legal troubles to keep his inventions off the market, she wanted all of us to go to Argentina to live. She believed that Rife could pursue his work there without interference or fear of the AMA or anyone else," Cleveland said, adding, "and looking back on it, we should have taken the advice."

"We thank you very much for letting us come. I hope you don't mind if we call you again, or come back as we proceed with this investigation," Herb said. Anjie nodded in agreement.

"Remember what I suggested. Forget about Rife and all this. Go back to Canada. Destroy those things and try to forget all of this," Cleveland said.

"Is that what you did?" Anjie asked, "try to forget. Did you succeed?"

"I did not. But I stayed alive," he whispered.

————

Anjie and Herb slumped back into the limo. "I wouldn't worry too much about what Cleveland said. He is an old man. I'm not sure how much we can believe of what he says," Herb said.

"I'm not a conspiracy freak of any kind but since you jeopardized our safety by talking about this all over the East Coast, I think we should at least be careful," Anjie said. She sits up and looks right into his eyes: "I don't mean to beat you to death over this, but we don't know what the people you talked to did with that information. Apparently it got to Cleveland. I just think we owe it to ourselves to proceed with caution."

"Are you having second thoughts now about this?"

"No. I am more enthusiastic than before we met Cleveland, but we must do some serious planning. If we're going to search for this Milhaus woman—every person we talk to about this will tell someone else. I think we need to understand there is danger-"

"-I am not taking it too seriously. This is old stuff. All that happened to Rife and his associates happened many years ago. We are not any threat to anyone," Herb said.

"No? Then you think it is all right with the pharmaceutical-medical complex now in this 21st Century, that we re-invent the Rife

84

instruments and end all diseases without drugs?" she asked, sarcastically.

"It all is so fanciful. I have difficulty believing it. I guess I don't want to believe that if such an invention existed, that someone or groups of powerful people would conspire to abolish it. Believing this is sort of like believing that the oil companies have a vested interest in keeping cars from running on water or something like that," he said testily.

"Well, don't you believe they do?"

———

"I checked with directory information for every city in southern California; there is no listing for Gertrude Milhaus. There are a few listings with that last name; I called them and no one knew Gertrude," Anjie said. "I'm drained, and at my wit's end for today."

Anjie and Herb are sitting at the table on the balcony of her suite looking into the darkness over the Pacific Ocean. "Don't worry about it. Why don't we go for a drink downstairs, and catch some of those sounds?," Herb asked. "You know the old saying about too much work and not enough fun…"

"I'm tired but you know, I do need a break. I rarely drink alcohol but tonight I am making an exception," she exclaimed. "I may even show you that I can dance-I guess- I call it dancing-and if they continue playing slow music, I will show you how; I am not such a cripple as you may think," she said, pulling herself up on her crutches. "That is, if you even want to dance with me!"

"Let's go before you change your mind."

The phone rings. Anjie reaches over to pick it up. "Yes, this is the woman who called about Gertrude Milhaus, but how do you know this?" Anjie motions for Herb. He pulls the chair out for her as she drops herself down into it. "Tonight? I guess so. Here at the hotel in the lobby? How will I know who you are? OK, one hour."

"That was Gertrude Milhaus!" Anjie exclaimed excitedly. "She is coming to the hotel; she is on the way. She will be here in less than an hour. She said she knows what we look like, not to worry," Anjie said. "She sounded very old."

"Now I am worried," Herb said, somewhat sarcastically.

8

"I'm disappointed," Anjie whispered. "Why would she call and not show up?"

"Anything can happen out there on the freeways. She did call you from a cell phone, didn't she?" Herb asked, leaning over on the lobby sofa, closer to Anjie.

"I don't know. She said she was on the way. I guess so. She said she would be here in less than an hour, and here it is two hours later-"

"-It is still a mystery as to how she knew where we were staying and how to reach us," Anjie said. "I should have asked her."

"That's simple. It had to have been Dr. Cleveland who contacted her. He told us he didn't know where she was, but he did that out of caution, just in case she would not agree to see us," Herb said, impatiently. "Who else could it be?"

"It could be one of the persons I spoke with on the phone. I called every Milhaus listed. I don't know, maybe she was even at one of those places."

It was nearly midnight but the lobby of the Del Coronado was full of people. "I guess I missed my big opportunity to dance with you," Anjie said, smiling. "Gertrude ruined our plans."

"It is never too late," Herb said, getting up off the sofa, offering his hands of support to Anjie. She accepted his help but rejected the idea of dancing. "I'm too emotionally spent right now. I got pretty high with expectations while waiting for Gertrude, but now I have this big disappointment to deal with. Maybe tomorrow," she said.

"In the morning we call Dr. Cleveland. Perhaps we can persuade him to give us Gertrude's phone number," Herb said. "I think she must have gotten cold feet, or it could be a flat tire or car trouble, virtually anything and guessing wont help."

Anjie and Herb were silent up the elevator to their floor. Anjie handed Herb the key to her suite. He opened it. She went through the door, turning around to see Herb standing back as though unsure whether he should go in or not. "I know it's late. But I could use some company," she said. The voice she heard was her voice, but she couldn't believe the words were. Suddenly she blushed in embarrassment.

———

It was nearly 8:30 when the phone rang, jolting Anjie awake. It was Herb. Was she up and ready?, he wanted to know. "Ready for what?," she asked. Herb suggested they have breakfast in her room, and then call Dr. Cleveland at the home. "Don't you dare show up for at least thirty minutes. Go ahead and order for us as it takes them that long," she said. "Order me a pot of coffee," she ordered.

Anjie had a hangover, the first one she ever had in her life. Herb introduced her to champagne; she loved it. She even bragged that 'it does not taste like liquor'. She remembered dancing with Herb a little, snuggling up to him on the sofa. They necked but they stopped short of any sexual contact. She was pretty sure of that, but the more she thought about it, the more she wondered. Was he doing more than just embracing her? Should she be so embarrassed that she can't discuss the evening with Herb? Or should she just forget about it, pretending it did not happen?

Herb arrived just as the food did. Other than small talk about the weather, the birds trying to land on the balcony, and the color of the ocean, they avoided discussion of Rife, his inventions, Dr. Cleveland, Gertrude Milhaus and even their late evening together, until Herb decided to bring it up. "I don't know whether to thank you or apologize for what happened last night," he said, eyes down. "I just don't know how you feel about it."

Anjie was tempted to ignore the comment but didn't. "I enjoyed it. Maybe I liked the champagne too much," she chuckled, "but I had fun and to be honest with you, it was the first time I remember ever feeling the way I did - I realize I probably shouldn't tell you this."

Exhaling, Herb drops back in his chair. "I couldn't sleep worrying about it. I mean-I thought I behaved myself, but I worried that I went beyond what you would approve of-'.

"-I guess I am a prude compared to other women you know. I think I probably overdue the prude thing but it is a habit, and sort of a self-defense mechanism that I developed to shield me from hurt. An attractive woman who happens to be handicapped gets used to men liking the way they look, until they find out that the handicap is permanent - so up goes a shield to protect us," she said. "I think you understand."

"Forget about that. In fact, let's forget about the whole thing, if it offends you at all," he said, emphatically.

"No, I don't want to forget it."

"Great! Let's call Dr. Cleveland about Gertrude Milhaus. Maybe we can convince him to help us get in contact with her," he said.

Anjie picked up the phone, glancing down at her notebook. She dialed the number at the nursing home. He did not answer but his voice mail did. She left a message. "Why don't you call the office, maybe they can page him or tell you where he is," he suggested. She did it.

"Cleveland left this morning about 8:00 o'clock in the company of a man and a woman. They said he is required to sign out and he did, estimating his return about 4:00pm this afternoon," she said.

"You mean he can just get up and go whenever he feels like it?"

"Of course." The woman hangs up.

"Yes, I remember, he said so himself yesterday. He is not under constant care. He still has freedom of movement. We can find something else to do in the meantime. We can wait and call him later."

"True. Also, you can call back all those Milhauses you called yesterday. Who knows, maybe Gertrude will answer the phone!"

"Good idea!"

———

"I've been calling for Dr. Cleveland all day. I was told he was expected about 4:00pm, but it is nearly seven and he still does not answer his phone. Do you know if he is in the building?" Anjie asked, anxiously. The voice on the end assured her that they have her message but that Dr. Cleveland has not returned. "Are you concerned that he has not returned?" The voice reminded Anjie that Cleveland was a 'guest' in the home and not a prisoner. He did not have to tell them anything about his whereabouts. "But you have a sign in and sign out form there. Isn't that required?" It is a courtesy form only. If he does not return by morning, there will be a reason for concern but as of now, there is not.

This bothered Anjie and Herb. The telephone calls to the Milhauses also failed. In fact, one of the numbers Anjie had reached yesterday was now disconnected.

"I don't want to get paranoid but maybe it is time?," she said.

"I agree. Why don't you relax a while? I'm going to my room to make some personal calls, and to follow up with some things. I am going to talk with one of our senior partners to see what advice he has to offer. I don't know what else to do," he said.

"Call from here. The way I feel right now, I really don't want you to leave," she said.

"Oh, look, we have nothing to fear. The old man may have some friends who take him out for a couple of meals and a long ride every now and then-"

"-What about the disconnected number?"

"Coincidence. Let's not start speculating, as we may conjure up all sorts of things that are not true. Going by what we know, there is no reason to worry about anything, at this point. But I'll call from here, if it makes you feel better."

———

The phone is ringing in a very large office in the law firm's building at Prince Edward Island. Bob Simpson, a longhaired, youthful black man is sitting across the desk reviewing a folder. Another man, Tony Pecoro, is sitting opposite, behind the desk. Pecoro, well dressed but unshaven and looking weary, is portly and somewhat frustrated. "Answer the fucking phone," he yells, looking up from some papers stacked in front of him. "Answer the phone!"

"Mr. Pecoro's office."

"Who is this?"

"Simpson."

"This is Herb Goldman, Bob. I know it is late but is Tony there?'

A pause and then an answer. "No, I'm sorry, he's not here. I think he is meeting his wife for dinner tonight."

"May I help you? Are you at the New York office? I haven't seen you in a few days."

"No, out in San Diego on personal business. I don't think you can help, unless you can tell me whether a check for $50,000 US was sent out here via FedEx. Do you know anything about it?"

"A check for $50,000?" Pecoro is nodding his head affirmatively. "Herb, yes, I am pretty sure that went out. You should have it tomorrow or the next day. Any message for Tony?"

"I wanted to discuss our client with him, Ms Anjanette de la Houssaye. As head of security for the firm, I think I need his advice. Will he be there in the morning?"

"Sure. I am looking at his calendar right now. Shall I have him call you?"

"No, we will call him. I don't know exactly what our schedule is tomorrow."

"Fine. Look, it is pretty damn late up here. I need to get home myself, before my wife comes up here to get me!," he chuckles.

"Sure. Thanks. Bye."

"You handled that well. I'm not ready yet to talk to him. When Cleveland doesn't show up again, and they can't find Gertrude

93

Milhaus, then he will need my help. That's when they will be right where we want them."

Simpson agreed. "What about our people at the nursing home?"

"Look, I like Goldman-have nothing against him- but you know, with this type of thing, we must be brutal. We have no choice. He is the lowest attorney on the totem pole here, with the most important client in the world. He was handling a probate for her, and fell into this other situation about the invention that supposedly cured cancer back in the thirties. That's why we were brought into this. As long as we can call the shots from PEI, we are in the clear. We must scrupulously avoid any tie-in to this firm with the actions we are forced to take down there."

"Especially this firm," Simpson said, "virtually all of our clients are international pharmaceutical companies, health insurance providers and research hospitals."

"I know. I got an initial report from our people in San Diego. Cleveland is gone, never again to be found by Goldman or his new best friend. As for Milhaus—we had that taken care of last night. As soon as Cleveland contacted her, we knew—she is also out of sight. The only thing bothering me is to what extant will Goldman go to find out what happened to them-," Pecoro said.

"-Forget that, he won't do anything. For one thing, he doesn't have the time; he has to come back here for work in a few days, and why should he? He doesn't really believe these instruments he found in the storage can do anything. As far as he is concerned, it is a pile of junk locked up in a dusty old barn, left there by some old screwball scientists and engineers. My guess is he is on this mission to get into the pants of the broad!," Simpson said.

Pecoro laughed, "I hope you are right. I wouldn't mind that either. She is one great looking woman."

"For what we are being paid to handle this, we must be right. When all this is over, we are multi-millionaires and certain senior partners in this firm will be worth hundreds of millions of dollars. That's what I think," Pecoro said.

"We must be tight. If we get one leak, if even one person finds out what is going on, we will have to line them up with their wives and husbands and kill them. What choice will we have?," Pecoro asked.

"I hope that doesn't happen but if it does, we will be there to do what we have to do," Simpson said. "Why do we have to handle it like this? Why cant we just go over to the storage locker, grab that stuff and dump it in the bay?"

"Because de la Houssaye has the diary and notebooks that were there, and Goldman has the engineering specs in safekeeping somewhere, and we don't know where. As long as we do not have that, even if the parts were destroyed—theoretically, the instruments can be redesigned and assembled. Until we have the whole package, we need to proceed with caution," Pecoro said. "And I mean c-a-u-t-i-o-n."

"You heard my end of the call, at least the advance of $50,000 is on the way to you. That will help you," Herb said.

"Right. Why does a law firm in PEI have a 'head of security'? I find that strange."

"You don't understand how large this firm is. We have over 1,500 attorneys in this law firm. Our head offices are in London and New York. We also have a very large office in Toronto with smaller ones in Paris and Rio de Janeiro-," he explained.

"Why PEI?"

"What you saw in PEI is somewhat of a deception. The firm only has a handful of lawyers there, nearly all of us associates—not partners. There is a junior partner responsible, but she doesn't even live at PEI. She comes in from Toronto."

"But all those people in that building? They all were working for the law firm, I saw that myself. I saw no other names anywhere."

"True but the firm uses PEI as its accounting processing location. All the accounting for the entire firm is done at PEI. Some years ago they got a special tax break, and other incentives to set that up, and that's what they did. I think they only paid $100 for the building! Of course, it was a mess and had to be renovated, but that was part of the deal. The head of security is in charge of the safety of all accounting and legal documents, as well as providing physical security when necessary to attorneys, who may need it from time to time."

"Why would an attorney need security?"

"Controversial cases, hard-fought ones that were many years old sometimes get settled in our favor and the losers—you get the idea," he shrugged. "They threaten the firm or the lawyers and we guarantee safety for them and their families."

"Why couldn't I have gone to Toronto instead of PEI?"

"Actually, we have an office in Vancouver, but you had to come to PEI because that is where the probate took place, and of course, where the property is located," he said.

Anjie shrugged. "I think we've had enough today. I'm tired and frustrated."

Herb agreed. "I'm leaving. I'm sorry but we seem to spin our wheels more than anything else. Tomorrow is another day." Herb leans over and holds Anjie tightly. She kisses him gently on the lips, and then eases out of his arms.

9

The bright orange rays of the rising sun dramatically illuminate the enormous sailing boats. In accelerated motion the sun travels across the sky. The beauty of the sunrise fascinates Anjie as she sips a cup of coffee, and stares out over the horizon. As early as it is this morning, she is surprised at the activity at the hotel restaurant below, and all the bodies already sunbathing in the distant sand. She did not sleep well, and is having second thoughts about what she and Herb are struggling to do in San Diego.

Anjie was never without money but she had very little. Her mother did the best she could. She may have been considered poor as a young child, but she didn't know she was poor, and really never thought about it. She reaches into her purse to remove her wallet. She pops out a warn photo of her mother. Anjie is wishing her mother were alive to advise her now, and to share with her their good fortune. Now that she soon will have over a million dollars in cash, plus her property in PEI, why doesn't she just go home? She can give notice properly at the newspaper, and vacate her apartment for more luxurious surroundings, either in the Vancouver area or in California or even Florida. If it is dangerous trying to reassemble those Rife instruments, why should she risk her life at a time when she has the money to enjoy it?

The ringing of the phone interrupts Anjie's thoughts. "Hello. Yes, this is Anjie de la Houssaye. There is a long pause. "Police? But I don't know anything about Dr. Cleveland. I only met him one time. It is true that I have been calling him, and leaving messages, but that is because I do not know where he is, and I was hoping to see him again."

The sheriff's office is calling as a result of a report from the nursing home that Dr. Cleveland left and never returned. A couple of the employees at the home told the police that the old man left with a young couple, and that he seemed happy when he was signing out. He told them, they said, he was going to visit an old friend. The officer asked if Anjie could meet him at the nursing home later in the morning. Of course, she said yes.

Advising Herb of the call was not so easy. He didn't answer his phone. Anjie had him paged in the lobby and restaurant but there were no responses. Suddenly she was full with emotions, the first being fear, and the second being jealousy. Was he in any danger? Or did he slip out last night to meet Sudsy at the all night joint? It was nearly thirty minutes before she got her answer; he showed up at the door dressed in a jogging suit.

"Good morning," he said cheerily. "Thought I would let you sleep-in this morning. I went for a run alongside the ocean. It was great," he said. "How are you this morning?"

"Not too good. For one thing, I was worrying about you, and I had a call from the police—sheriff's office, really-and they want us to meet them at the nursing home. Cleveland didn't return from his outing, and they want to talk to us about it."

"Give me a few minutes to clean up and I will meet you here," he gasped.

"Why don't we just meet in the lobby?"

"OK, are you calling the limo service for the car?"

"No, I am calling the driver, Wolfgang, direct. He gave me his card."

———

"So far, two of the employees we interviewed here at the home told us that Cleveland left here with you. How do you account for that?," the deputy asked, flipping a notebook in his hand. "Why would they say that, if it were not true?"

Herb and Anjie stared at each other in disbelief. The deputy seemed old for the job but he was friendly. Herb did not want a confrontation. "I am an attorney. I am telling you that we came here to see him and he was gone. A receptionist told us he signed out with a man and a woman; she told us he would be back that afternoon. We called and he was still not back. This is all we know," Herb said, restraining his growing anger. "I have no idea how they got us mixed up with that couple. Cleveland certainly did not leave here with us."

"Strange," the deputy said, slowly nodding his head negatively, "very strange. The employees are positively certain it was you, but let's leave that for a while. What is your relationship to Cleveland?"

"Relationship? None. We just met him," Anjie responded.

"What is your business with Cleveland?"

The question Herb dreaded the most. "We have no business with him. He was a research scientist on a project from many years ago. We just wanted to meet him; we may write about him."

"And then what?"

"Nothing. Meet him—we are in San Diego and thought it was a good idea," Herb said, not very convincingly.

"Officer, we want to find him as much as you do. That's why we've been calling him on the phone," Anjie said, obviously frustrated.

"All that calling on the phone—some folks might think that is to establish an alibi or something," he said, matter-of-factly. "But you know how suspicious cops are, since you are an attorney," the deputy said. "And you, Miss, what do you do?"

"I am the editor of a newspaper in Canada," she said confidently. "I am a reporter."

"Then you are working on a story down here?"

"Yes, that's right."

"And your newspaper publisher will verify this?"

Seeing the uncertainty in Anjie's eyes, Herb answered. "That is neither here nor there. She does not need to prove anything to anyone. She told you, she is a reporter."

"Sir, I don't disbelieve her. She is a reporter working on a story. What is the story?"

"This is ridiculous," Herb said. "She doesn't have to answer these questions. And unless you have a reason to hold us here, we're leaving," he said firmly. "We can be reached at the Del Coronado Hotel."

Herb nudges Anjie to start walking. She does a few steps, and then stops. "Officer, I think you better find out why those employees are not telling the truth. They know we are not the couple Cleveland left with. I can assure you of that."

"Lady, those employees have been here a long time, and they are local residents of this community, with clean records. They are not the ones from out of town traveling in limousines," he retorted.

Herb looked at Anjie intently. "Enough. Let's get out of here."

"Wait—hold up there, you two. Give me your passports. We will give them back after we checked you out. In the meantime, do not leave the hotel until you've heard from us," the old deputy's demeanor had changed. He was no longer a friendly old man, but an angry law enforcement officer.

"Anjie hands her passport over to the old deputy. "I'm an American citizen residing in Canada on a permit." Herb hands the document over.

"We'll be in touch," he said. "You can go".

———

Anjie and Herb finally see the luxury yacht harbored at San Diego with the name "Prescription." Many people are walking about the boat, many in bathing suits; some are dancing. A few are making love. A loud Jamaican band is adding to the festivities. Waitresses costumed as nurses and doctors are fielding bumps and grinds from guests, who are playfully trying to spill the champagne or knock over the caviar. The yacht belongs to the head of a large firm, and this is his party. The man, Turner von Atziger, is standing with his arms around two young women wearing bikinis. His shirt is off but he is wearing powder blue trousers, and a yachtsman's cap. He spots Anjie and Herb on the shore; he is waving to them. "Welcome aboard! Come on up," he orders.

Anjie is intimidated by the high incline of the gangway. Herb senses this. Without her permission or further discussion, he reaches down and picks her up until he has her body on both arms. She objects but he manages to reach the deck with only a gasp for air. Gently he turns her over and stands her on her feet. "Bet you didn't think I could do that," he grinned.

Anjie's eyes are moving through the people on the boat; some are flirting, and others are well on the way to being drunk. She is asking herself, why am I here? As Turner approaches to welcome them, she sees a man emerge from below deck, but his back is to them, looking the opposite way. Unlike the others, he is wearing a suit and carrying an attaché case.

"Welcome! You are Anjie and Herb?" They nod agreement. "Good. Tony Pecoro told me what is going on; he asked me to help. We are long-term friends and clients of the firm, and since I stay in San Diego six months a year, he immediately thought I was the best person to assist you."

Turner is sixtyish but appears younger as a result of cosmetic surgery. He is suntanned and tall with flowing white hair. He has deep blue eyes. He speaks with a French accent. He excuses the two girls on his arms, neither of which can be older than 17 or 18. Anjie had persuaded Herb to call Pecoro for advice, and now it is their obligation to follow it. The advice was to see Turner for help. Now, here they were, and Anjie didn't like it.

"Over here. We'll have some privacy," Turner said. A cabin door opens and the man with the suit and attaché was there, nudging Anjie and Herb to attention. The man with the suit is introduced only as "Charles." The man is so big that he blocks the vision of the rest of the cabin that appears very small. A strange orange light pervades in the room. "We could go below deck, but I am afraid that all the cabins are in use now," Turner said, chuckling. "This is a storage room but it will do. We wont be here long."

Instead of deck mops and cleaning equipment, the room was full of shelves with maps. Charles opens his briefcase and hands Herb a pistol. "What is that?," asked Anjie, anxiously. "Why are you giving him a gun?"

"It is a .357 Magnum. Just point it and pull the trigger. The assailant will stop and drop to the ground," Charles said. "It is part of what you need to be safe out here, if what Tony told us is true."

Herb accepts the weapon but examines it closely. He notices it is not loaded. "Oh, yea, here is a box of shells," Charles says, after fishing the shell box from his attaché. "You can't buy a gun in California, this is why Tony asked us to get you one. It's clean."

Anjie objects. "I'm not against guns, but for us to have one, I think it is dangerous. What if the police find it on us?"

"You can't let that happen. Keep it in your room when you are there, or in your car, just don't ever carry it. You'll be OK," Charles assured them.

"Is this what your firm calls help?," Anjie asked, nervously jabbing Herb's arm. "I thought he was giving us private detective assistance!"

"He is," Turner said, "that is why Charles is here. He is going to investigate the disappearance of this Dr. Cleveland, and also find Gertrude Milhaus for you. These are the things you need done. Right?"

"Well, yes, but one more thing: Two employees at the home identified us as the couple Dr. Cleveland left the home with and this is ridiculous. We don't understand how that could happen. They know damn well it is not us," Anjie said, excitedly. "I am very suspicious as to how this ended up like this."

"And with good reason," Turner said. "Well, look, Charles has the info and your contact numbers. He will get started right away. He will be in touch with you-"

"-How do we get in touch with Charles?," Anjie asked.

"You don't," Charles said, "and this is for your own safety. We want to avoid any connection together."

"Good. This is all done and now I can get back to my party. We have an interesting couple of days ahead," Turner said.

———

Uneasy and unsure of the propriety of what they were doing, and feeling very uneasy about this connection with the mysterious Charles, Anjie worried aloud about Charles running around searching for Dr. Cleveland and Milhaus. In the limo en route back to the hotel in Coronado, Anjie lowers the partition window to ask Wolfgang a question. Herb seems surprised and angered by it.

"Wolfgang, do you work for the law firm?"

"No, I work for a company owned by the firm."

"Oh, so that is why they contacted you about me coming down to San Diego and Mr. Goldman?"

"Yes, that's right. They sent a message to our office; I was assigned."

"Do you know the owner of that yacht we just left?"

"Yes, I know him. We drive him, also, when he and his staff are in town."

"What does he do for a living?"

Wolfgang pauses. "I'm not sure. I don't think anyone ever said." Anjie feels Wolfgang is holding back.

"But he told us he was a major client of the law firm—"

"-Perhaps that is true but I have no way of knowing things like that. They don't tell me. I'm just a driver," he chuckled, glancing back to Herb Goldman.

"I think you are badgering poor Wolfgang and he is busy driving, Anjie. He doesn't know anything."

"Do you?"

"Very little. Stuck up at PEI, we are not really privy to insider information. I don't know one client from another," he said.

Anjie felt very much ill at ease. "Herb, did you notice the medical theme of that party?"

"Yes, nurses in short costumes with low cut tops-that is a favorite fantasy of every man-"

"-And is taking prescription drugs also a favorite fantasy?"

"Why do you ask that, Anjie?"

"The name of the yacht: 'Prescription?'" "These people are in the pharmaceutical or medical business. They must be!"

"Our firm handles all sorts of clients. Some of them are in that business."

"And we are accepting help from them? Are we crazy?"

Wolfgang raises the petition.

Herb doesn't answer. He merely looked out the window and nodded his head negatively.

―――

Rev. Harry Fine, perhaps 40, is the charismatic leader of the congregation where Anjie worships. With a twinkle in his eye and a sharp-gaze, he gives off a decidedly non-religious aura. He has wide shoulders and an athletic presence that remind everyone he once played professional football in the United States. He is standing alone in his office talking on the telephone to Anjie. He is tall and massive, looking more like a wrestler than a preacher. Anjie respects his opinion, and often discusses personal issues with him. At one time, she admits to having a crush on Fine, but he never reciprocated any interest. Some women in the congregation have speculated as to his sexual preference, as several of the women failed at arousing his interest. The fact that he shares his home with a young Asian man who is his assistant, only invites further speculation. Tonight she is calling from San Diego, where she is troubled by the events of the last few days.

His finely etched facial features give way to concern as he listens. "Anjie, from what you have told me, you are placing yourself more and more in danger every day. You need help, and it doesn't sound to me like this guy Charles is the answer. If his solution is to give you a gun, then I must question what skills he has."

Fine sits down and begins writing notes on a legal pad. "Stop. I don't think you should tell me all the details. I am happy for you as far as the inheritance is concerned, but all the money in the world can't save you from evil. If these people have spent the last sixty or so years suppressing this invention, they are not going to stop now. Frankly, I think you should be talking with the FBI."

Fine writes notes with a furious pace and then drops the pencil down. "Anjie, you are repeating yourself. Either you call the FBI or let me do it for you. And as far as this guy GOLD-MAN, I wouldn't trust him any further than you can see him. Remember, he works for these people."

Fine is what is called by some Christians a 'completed' Jew-a Jew who converted to Christianity. Other Jews have much harsher names for those who make this conversion. Fine reminds Anjie. "You know you have to consider what you are dealing with. This is a law firm with close ties to the pharmaceutical and medical industries, the very same groups that will do anything to prevent you from reinventing that Rife instrument. You are not in friendly country," he said.

He listens and then doodles, drawing little pictures of crosses on the pad. "Would you like for me to come down there? If there is ever a time when you need support, it is now. And since you can afford to pay my expenses, I am willing to accept the challenge! I don't like what you are facing down there."

There is a long pause. "Excellent. Don't tell your GOLD-MAN I am coming. We will make it look like it is purely coincidental. Give me your cell number, I will call back with the arrival information." A long pause. "Don't worry. I wont stay at the same hotel. This must look purely coincidental."

Fine hangs up, leaning back in his chair, smiling. He appears very contented.

10

A black man in a well-tailored business suit exits from a taxi in front of Marie Callender's Restaurant in Coronado. He pays the taxi while checking his watch. Anjie, inside the restaurant at a window table, eyes the man carefully. She follows him as he walks into the restaurant carrying a small briefcase. He wears a little smile on his face and appears friendly. He either says hello or nods positively to everyone he sees. Without looking around the restaurant to find Anjie, he sits at the counter and orders a coffee. Anjie is disappointed that he is not the FBI agent who is supposed to meet her.

Just as she is verifying the time on her watch, a man about thirty-five enters the restaurant, immediately joining Anjie, as though he knew her. He is David Hillyer of the FBI. He does not know Anjie, but he knew whom to look for. He spotted the "Madeline Stowe" look-a-like immediately, he said.

Hillyer has the well-groomed appearance expected of the FBI, but his face is lined with boredom or bitterness. He is unhappy about his life or assignment; he has very little interest in what Anjie has to say. He wants to be somewhere else. Although wearing an expensive dark suit, Anjie notes it is ill fitting with his sleeves a little too long, and the shoulders droopy. Anjie is thinking this is a man who has lost a lot of weight!

The waitress knows him. "Coffee, with a piece of apple pie?," she says cheerily. "And you? What would you like?"

"Coffee. Black."

The young waitress quickly turns away. Hillyer nods goodbye to the girl, as he observes her wiggling away. He is obviously admiring her rear-end! Anjie tries to knock him back to reality. "Are you Hillyer, the FBI agent?"

He doesn't answer; instead, he sizes up Anjie. "You do look like Madeline Stowe," he says. "You were easy to find."

"I'm not lost, Agent Hillyer. I need help but I'm not lost!," she declared.

"Tell me about it."

Anjie, very slowly and methodically, in sequential order, relayed the entire story from the time she arrived at PEI, up until her phone conversation with Rev. Fine last night. She stresses the need for the utmost of secrecy. While she tells the story, Hillyer appears disinterested, even distracted by people filling the sidewalks across the street at the boutiques, and following the women with interest. Anjie, however, never stops talking until she has the entire story told. She is frustrated; already convinced she is wasting her time. She regrets going behind Herb's back to follow Fine's advice about talking to the FBI.

Hillyer motions impatiently to the sexy waitress he likes; he complains good-naturedly that it is taking too long for their order. She says nothing but smiles; she returns promptly with a tray. She has both orders. He thanks her. Once again he watches her as she struts away. "Did you hear anything that I told you?," Anjie asked, impatiently.

"Everything. There is no federal crime committed that we know of, so far, so there is little we can do except make a report on it and then, if anything arises, we will have this background information on file," he says, sipping his coffee slowly. "We do not have evidence of any crime and it does not seem that you do, either," he said.

"We have two people missing," Anjie retorted. "I am from Canada where it is a federal crime to kidnap people, and as far as I know, it is a crime in the USA, also," she says, impatiently. Hillyer says nothing, choosing instead to eat his pie.

"I heard what you said about the persons you think are missing. Before coming out here, I checked the computer, and there is NO missing person report filed on either Cleveland or Milhaus. They are the persons you told me on the phone are missing. Isn't that correct?"

"Yes. I was at the nursing home where Cleveland lives, and the deputy sheriff was there, investigating. He must have filed a report."

"Maybe he did file a report, internally, but this guy has not been missing long enough yet to file a missing person report on him. And we have no reports at all on the woman, Gertrude-"

"-I just gave you a report. They are both missing-"

"-You told me on the phone you do not even know the woman, and only met the old man once. You are not a relative or even a friend or acquaintance—there is no way your report can move the bureau," he said emphatically, returning to his pie.

"Can you stop eating long enough to look and listen to me?"

Surprised, and teased, Hillyer puts the fork down. He leans forward toward Anjie. "I heard everything you said. As far as that invention is concerned, we know nothing about that, and will have nothing to do with that aspect of this unless you or someone has evidence of a federal law being violated. This is what we will do: I will go back to the office and 302 this information. My supervisor will read it, and so will his supervisor read it. Who knows how high it will go? IF-and I say IF-anyone believes an investigation should follow, I will get back to you."

"How long will that take?"

"Who knows?"

"I am risking a lot sitting her talking to you. The lawyer from the firm, Herb Goldman—he thinks I am having physical therapy- if he knew I was talking to the FBI, I don't know what he would do or say," she said. "I plead with you. PLEASE do something to help find out what happened to these people!"

In a more understanding and conciliatory tone, Hillyer promises that he will "snoop around" a little, but that he does not have the authority to do more than that. "The employees you told me about at the nursing home, which identified you and Goldman as the couple who drove off with Cleveland, do you have their names?"

"I'm sorry, no, I don't have them. The sheriff's deputy who was at the home investigating knows who they are. He was the one who told me about them identifying us."

Hillyer threw a $10 bill on the table. He leaned over to Anjie. "Physical therapy? Those are your crutches, obviously; what is the problem?"

"Oh, I had an accident. I'm supposed to have physical therapy at least twice a week," she said, as though it was not that important. "I used it as an excuse."

"Do you need some help getting out of here?"

"No, thanks. I am going to shop up the street a few minutes before returning to the Del."

"Lady, if there is any truth at all to what you have told me, it would be wise for you to get out of here. Have you considered going back to Canada?"

"The sheriff has my passport; he told me not to leave," she said, flippantly.

"Aha, aha. Well, be careful. IF I find out anything, I will call you. If you find out anything, call me!"

The sexy waitress spotted Hillyer leaving; she hurried over to him. They spoke briefly. She returned to the table to pick up the $10 bill. "Anything else, for you?"

"I'm finished. No thank you," she said. "I'm finished."

As Anjie is getting up to leave, the black man she first observed earlier at the counter came over. "I see you have crutches; please allow me to assist you," he says, holding a crutch in one hand while boosting Anjie with the other.

"Oh, that is not necessary, but thank you. I can manage," she said, gratefully. "It is nice of you, but I do not need any help."

He leaned over and whispered in her ear. "You may need my help. That's why I'm here. I saw you out at the yacht. We've had you under observation ever since then," he said. "Suggest we sit down and chat. I can help you a lot more than that FBI agent can. Take my word for it."

Anjie was not afraid of him, but she was apprehensive, surprised and worried. She dropped back down in the booth. He took the crutches and leaned them gently against the booth. "Now, let's get to the bottom of this," he said, calmly.

"Lip readers have a decided advantage," he said. "I could see everything you said in that mirror over there, and some of what he said. It is special training that comes in handy," he grinned.

The sexy waitress returns, perplexed but pleasant. He hands her a $10 bill and tells her to leave them alone. She smiles and does exactly that. Anjie notices that this man does not watch the waitress as she struts away. She likes that. She stares back at the man in pensive puzzlement, waiting for him to tell why he is there. Finally, he smiles, saying there is nothing to be concerned about, as far as he is involved; he is a friend.

"My name is Joe Smith. I am with Interpol. That is about all you need to know about me at this time. We have an active investigation involving persons who were on that yacht; we want to know all about why you were there with your companion. What can you tell me?"

"Joe Smith? What a joke. Interpol? Prove it," Anjie orders, rudely.

He reaches inside his jacket pocket to remove a portfolio. He hands it to her. Anjie opens it. "You are Joe Smith. I am assuming this is an alias," she smiles.

"You are wrong. Joe Smith is my name, but we are not here to talk about me. Remember, I overheard all that you and the FBI agent spoke about. Now I want to know what is your connection with the people on that yacht?"

"None. The owner of the yacht, Turner—he is a client of this law firm that my companion works for—and he happened to be in town, so we were invited. I got out there and didn't feel well, so we left," she lied.

"How well do you know Turner?"

"I don't know him at all."

"And Charles Robertson?"

"Never heard of him!"

"You met with him on the yacht. He had his brief case with him."

117

"Oh, I just met him, that's all."

"Ms de la Houssaye, I am afraid that you are searching for trouble. You need a private detective and Charles is sent to you by the firm—"

"OK, what do you want from me? We asked him to help us find these missing persons," she explained.

"This business about the missing persons. Does this have anything to do with Turner von Atziger or any of his associates?"

"None. That is another problem unrelated to anything else. As for Turner—from what I heard and saw, he is a very wealthy international business man; what can be wrong with that?"

"A lot can be wrong with it. Do you know Tony Pecoro?"

"Only from what Herb Goldman told me. He is the head of security for the firm."

"He has an assistant by the name of Bob Simpson, a black guy; did you meet him in Canada?"

"No, I don't know anything about him."

"These are bad eggs. They're up to their elbows in shady dealings all over the world. If they get involved with what you are doing here, call me immediately." He hands Anjie a business card. She drops it in her purse.

"We ran a background check on you—you came up clean. My advice is that if you want to stay that way, is to stop associating with these characters you are encountering down here. It may also be a good idea to forget about that invention. That is ancient history. I can get your passport back from the sheriff, but only if you return home, and forget about all this—"

"-I can't do that."

"Another thing. This companion of yours, Goldman-I read what you were saying-let me tell you that the firm he works for has 3,500 employees, many of them lawyers and lobbyists. Their specialty is representing the largest pharmaceutical and medical complexes in the world. Goldman works for them. I don't know what he is telling you, but believe this-he knows what goes on in that firm, and who their clients are-if I were you, I would not trust him."

"I don't know whether he is honest with me or not," Anjie said, sadly.

"Then all I can tell you is be careful," he warned.

———

Across a small living room full of suitcases and boxes, Sudsy Lanahan, a raw, sexy woman, stands in her panties and bra. She is upset about something, yanking files out of boxes, putting them on a living room table. Finally she finds the one file she needs. "I have it, at last; if you want to go through it, do it now while I get dressed." She seems to be talking to the wall, as there is no one else in the room. The only other sounds being music from a small transistor radio on the floor.

Sudsy leaves the room. Just as she does, Herb Goldman enters, carrying two glasses of wine. He looks at the thick red file on the table, puts the wine down, taking the file in his hand. He sits on the only furniture in the room, one of the cheap folding chairs that came with the table. He rushes through the pages until he finds what he is looking for. "Laura, I found it. It's Tony Pecoro's report from when he interviewed you. He states right here that the firm agreed to pay $5,000 a week for a minimum of five weeks; provide a rental Mercedes for at least 90 days; all expenses; and $1,500 a month for rent." After pausing a while, he yells out: "Can you hear me, Laura?"

The woman rushes back in the room. This time she is dressed wearing only a bath robs. Her hair is wet. "I heard you. So? Where is the money? So far all I got was an advance of $3,000. This is bullshit. I want all the money at one time. This job is worth more than that. What if this 'Anjie' knew she didn't even inherit any land in San Diego, and that all of this is part of a scam to cheat her out of her inventions?" Herb says nothing. She glances down at the file and then at Herb. "This is the easiest acting job I've ever had!," she laughs. "I'm not threatening anyone. I've done a lot of things for money that I wouldn't tell my mother about, but I never made this kind of money. Call them and tell them to wire the funds tomorrow."

She pushes the table and file aside, attempting to sit on Goldman's knee, but the flimsy chair breaks, throwing both of them to the floor, laughing and hugging each other. Rolling over on his back, she climbs up on top of him, tickling him at the same time. "Stop! Stop! Come on Laura—come on—I'll call Pecoro in the morning."

They move rhythmically, kissing and touching. Goldman eases the robe off her body while holding her hair in his hands, drawing her body against his. Goldman turns her around to where he is on top. She urges him to get on with it. "Come on, come on…"

Finally, he pushes himself up. His head is resting on her chest. She holds him for a long time and then lowers herself against him once again. She kisses him gently on the lips and eyelids. She reaches below and tells him to do it again.

They make love again without speaking another word.

———

A pianist croons the last few bars of another Sinatra tune. A waiter, Pablo, shows the last two patrons to the door. Pablo and a woman, begin putting up chairs; the pianist, slips into a stool at the bar. Anjie is watching with interest. She doesn't ever recall being in a restaurant or bar when it was closing. "It is getting late, Harry, and I know you have to be tired from the trip down here. The airports are such a problem these days," she says sincerely. "By the way, you told me where to meet you tonight, but you didn't tell me what hotel you are in."

"I'm not in a hotel, Anjie. I have a buddy that I played football with in the NFL, some years ago. He is a high-flying financial consultant who lives in New York City most of the time, but he has a great condo in La Jolla. I am staying at his condo on the ocean. I drove here in his Porsche," he said, smiling. "I hope I don't get used to this extravagant lifestyle."

"You wont. Now that you know the whole story, what do you think I should do?"

"The important thing is your personal safety and the safe-keeping of that diary, those drawings and certainly, all those parts. It worries me that the people who know about this invention from firsthand experience are missing, after you contacted them. This indicates a possible problem for you-I wonder about the trustworthiness of GOLD-MAN."

"I think he can be trusted. He did not know that stuff was in the storage, until the same time I did. That's what convinces me he is probably straight—I mean, that he did not know in advance about any of it—so he couldn't have planned anything, such as helping me or coming down to San Diego with me. He and I saw it all for the first time in that storage unit together. But I must admit concern about the law firm that employs him. He didn't tell me that they are heavily involved with the pharmaceutical-medical complex, and frankly, that does bother me."

Harry holds Anjie's hand. "Don't worry. I am going to see what I can find out about this whole episode down here; but there is something I can do that is much more important to me-"

"-What is that?"

"Persuade you to leave that hotel. You can tell GOLD-MAN that you are taking a condo out at La Jolla. He can go or stay, whatever he wants to do. Tell him a friend up in Canada owns it, and you decided to use it while he is out of town."

"He can't do anything he wants to do, the sheriff's office has my passport and his Canadian Residency Card. Neither of us can leave until they tell us it is OK," she shrugged.

"Let him do what he wants. You come on out to La Jolla. My friend is in New York with no plans to come in." Anjie hesitates, once again eyeing the clean-up crew and the singer who is now drinking Margaritas at the bar.

"I'll check out tomorrow."

"Your driver—who is he?"

"Someone hired by the firm to drive us around."

"Then why isn't he driving GOLD-MAN tonight?"

"I don't know. I left with the limo, and have had it all day. Herb said he was going to take care of personal business today. I told him I was having physical therapy and shopping."

"Come back with me to La Jolla, and don't tell the driver where we're going. In fact, just tell him to go home. We'll pick up your stuff tomorrow, and check you out then," he urged.

"Are you that concerned for me?"

"Yes. Don't go back, and don't tell anyone where you are. Pick up the check," he said, grinning widely, "and we can go!"

Anjie's feelings for Rev. Harry Fine were always ambiguous. She was never sure whether she admired him for his work and commitment to the congregation and community, or because he is handsome, strong and gentle. Tonight, she is having that same mixed up feeling. Although Harry had two glasses of wine, Anjie had only one, so she did not attribute her ambiguity to the wine. There was, though, the possibility she was interested in leaving with Harry to see what will happen, if anything. Is this the night she finds out whether he is gay or not? She scorned herself for even thinking the thoughts.

"OK, let's go-"

"When we go out that door, we must look like a couple, not just friends. This driver has to think we have a connection going on-"

She laughs aloud. "Shame on you, Reverend!"

———

Wolfgang is on the cell phone talking when Anjie knocks on his window, startling him. He immediately disconnects. As soon as he was out the door, she told him to go ahead without her. Fine skips over and wraps his arms around her, smiling; he said nothing but kissed her on her neck. Obviously surprised, Wolfgang said, "If that is what you want, but I will be happy to drive you both where you are going. No trouble at all."

"It's not necessary," Harry says, joyfully, "as I got that new Porsche over there. I don't think this beautiful woman has ever had a ride in a Porsche."

"Where are you headed?," Wolfgang asked.

"I have a condo near here. We are going to party the rest of the night," he said, nudging Anjie to agree.

"Party? That's something I haven't done in a long while!," she said enthusiastically.

"Where do you live?"

Refusing to get upset at Wofgang's impertinence, Harry just smiled. "Let's go," he said. Without another word, Anjie and Harry left Wolfgang standing outside the limo watching them stroll away.

The sign welcoming visitors to La Jolla surprised Anjie. They had only been driving a few minutes. Harry said that he was very familiar with the city from his days when he played with the NFL San Diego Chargers. "It is a mini Beverly Hills, in many ways. The shopping here will test the limits of your credit card's patience and understanding, that is for sure," he laughed. "The beaches are great and for southern California, the restaurants are super fantastic. It is a very affluent area. Actually, there is somewhat of a European atmosphere, with great art galleries and many cultural attractions."

While uncomfortable in the Porsche, Anjie did not have the feeling of terror she had riding with Sudsy Lanahan to view the empty lot. She said nothing, preferring to enjoy the ride and company. To her surprise, she liked both.

The condo was more than spectacular. Six bedrooms and six baths, a view of the ocean and all the amenities one can imagine, including a built in sauna and training room. "What would a single man need with a place like this?," she asked. To her surprise, the owner of the condo paid about $2-million a few years ago, and he only recently turned down twice that amount, according to Harry. Some investment, she said.

Harry helped get her comfortable in the living room. Soon he returned with two glasses of wine. Anjie did not object. "I think you should call GOLD-MAN. Try to put him at ease. Tell him you are at a friend's condo and that you will see him tomorrow sometime. See if he has any news."

"OK." She picks up the phone, dialing Herb's cell phone number. Herb sits beside her. "Hi, this is Anjie-," she said, and then paused for quite a time. "I don't like hearing this but I guess we have no choice...I am at a friend's condo in San Diego somewhere.

...No, I think it is better if I just meet you at the hotel in the morning. I am going to check out of the Del to move in over here. We can go to the sheriff's office together to see what happens." She hangs up without another word.

Anjie looks intently at Harry. "He said we have to go to the sheriff's office tomorrow about the missing Dr. Cleveland and the woman, Gertrude Milhaus. They apparently are calling in the two employees from the nursing home to confront us, to see if they will agree they made a mistake or what."

"Good. I'm going with you."

"But why? How can I explain that?"

"Just tell them I am your friend and let it go at that."

"I'm scared, Harry, really scared." Anjie dropped her head onto his shoulder. He holds her tightly, and then they kiss, lightly. She buries her head in his broad chest while he strokes her hair. "I don't know how to react to this," she whispers.

"Just do what you feel comfortable doing. It is up to you," he said.

11

The door to the room opens and the bellman, followed by Herb Goldman, walks into the room. He puts Anjie's bags onto one of those huge luggage holders. "Anything else, mam?"

"No, thank you. I will follow you down in a few minutes," Anjie says. Goldman hands the man a $10 bill. He nods but says nothing. Goldman pulls the door shut after the bellman exits.

"What is this all about? Why is that guy with you?"

"Coincidence. He happened to be in San Diego the same time as we are. He is staying in this condo of a friend, and there is plenty of room, so I am moving over there," she says, trying to maintain a laid-back attitude about it all. In the meantime, she is checking all the draws and closets to be certain nothing is being left behind.

"I hope that you did not tell him anything about why we are here or the inventions or anything like that," he says, holding her with both hands. "Too many people already know about this." Goldman seems worried.

"Seems as though you are forgetting that it is I who inherited the papers, drawings, spec sheets and parts. I have an obligation, in my mind-a duty, really-to make the most of it that I can. This man is a minister and friend. I am glad he is here. I don't think you should be cautioning me about telling others; it was you who made the phone calls all over the East Coast that alerted everyone. And that law firm you work for, seems as though their interest is the exact opposite of mine."

Goldman stands back. Anjie pushes forward past him toward the door. "Look, I just wanted to help. The two of us are going to the sheriff's office, and we will get that over with—depending upon how that ends; I will then make arrangements to leave. I don't think I am serving any good purpose here any more," he said.

"I agree. I got the check for $50,000 yesterday. I opened an account here. When I get the proceeds from the sale of the San Diego property, I will reimburse you guys. I signed the note and documents. I shipped them back to Canada via FedEx."

"Oh, well, glad that is handled. Now you can pay your bill downstairs," he quipped. "Are we all riding out together in the limo or are you traveling by Porsche these days?"

"We are going to follow Wolfgang out there. How did you know about the Porsche?"

Looking a little befuddled, he replied: "I guess Wolfgang told me."

———

The sheriff's office is big, modern and surprisingly prosperous looking, located in an industrial area that is well landscaped. Anjie expected nothing like this. They are met by a receptionist behind a bulletproof glass who advises them to sit down, before she even inquires as to what is they want. From where they sit, they cannot see the office or other areas. In a few minutes, a young man appears from behind the locked door to ask if they would like something to drink. All three decline.

Once inside behind the door it appears chaotic. Rather than offices, most of the space is open, segmented only by portable low walls. Along the outer walls, below the long line of windows, is a shelf filled with three ring binders. They are escorted passed a large office with fifty or more persons working at computers, standing and talking or staring out at them, drinking coffee. Finally they reach the end of a corridor where the old deputy is standing outside a room. He grins but says nothing. He swings his arm toward the door; they follow their escort into the room. To their surprise, it is a media room. It appears to have TV, and electronic hookups, a very large drop down TV screen, and a small stage equipped with audio and video cameras. They are told to sit and wait.

"I don't like this," Goldman says. "I don't like the way this looks. Before you answer any questions about anything, consult with me.

Actually, it would have been a good idea to bring a local lawyer out here with us," he says, somewhat breathlessly.

"I'm not worried. This whole thing is a mistake," Anjie says. Harry Fine says nothing but he reaches over and takes Anjie's hand in his.

A few minutes later, two uniformed men and a woman rush into the room. "I'm sorry to keep you waiting," the woman says, "I'm Sheriff Johnson. We are here to tie up some reporting data about Dr. Cleveland, who is, reportedly, missing. We appreciate your help."

The Sheriff is attractive; she looks more like a model than a sheriff. Anjie couldn't hold back her curiosity about her. "Sheriff Johnson, please, may I ask you a question?"

"Of course," she smiled.

"How did you become a sheriff?"

Johnson laughs. "I was an FBI agent stationed here in San Diego County. I became well known as a result of a kidnapping case we had out here. Some people came to me-they asked me to run for office. I did and I won," she smiled.

"Amazing, thank you."

"And you are Anjanette de la Houssaye, a Canadian resident of British Columbia; one of you is Herb Goldman, an American citizen who is a resident of Prince Edward Island in Canada; and one of you is their lawyer. Right?"

They all laugh. "No, I am not a lawyer. I am a minister and friend of Ms de la Houssaye. I just came along for moral support, I guess. I don't really know what this is all about," he said.

"Then, sir, you should wait in the office across the corridor." Johnson turns to the old deputy. "Show this gentleman where he can wait; see that he is comfortable. Deputy, are your witnesses present?"

"Yes, Sheriff, they're here. They have been waiting in the back." He nods to Harry to follow him. Harry embraces and lightly kisses Anjie before leaving. Anjie smiles widely. Goldman's face is expressionless.

"Ms de la Houssaye and Mr. Goldman, please, stand over there under those lights. We have two employees from the nursing home who are being asked to take a look at you, so they can then tell us whether or not you are the folks they saw Dr. Cleveland leave the home with the other morning. Do you understand?"

"Yes, sheriff, we understand but this is ridiculous. We were not the couple!"

"Mr. Goldman, you are apparently an attorney, so you know that this is not an accusation of anything. We are conducting an investigation into this man's disappearance, if, indeed, he is even a missing person—this is one of the many actions we are required to take."

Goldman nods affirmatively. Anjie is already standing under the lights. The lights are so bright that when standing under them, the figures outside the platform cannot be made out in detail. When the two witnesses enter the room, their two forms could be seen moving around, but their features are not recognizable.

After about five minutes, Sheriff Johnson switches the lights off. "You can come off the platform now." Anjie gets down without any assistance. The two witnesses are gone.

"OK, this is where we stand with this as of now," Johnson said, in a very authoritative voice. "Ms de la Houssaye, you are positively identified as the female who accompanied Dr. Cleveland out of the building." She moves over to Goldman. "You are off the hook. They said that you are 'positively not' the man who was with Cleveland and the woman. You can go. We will have to ask Ms de la Houssaye to stay for further questioning."

"Go? Oh, no, I can't leave here without Anjie."

"Then we will find you a comfortable place to sit and wait. Perhaps you can join the Reverend across the hall," Johnson said, motioning for the old deputy to show Goldman the room. "Miss de la Houssaye, please come with us."

"May I stop to see Rev. Fine?"

"Of course." Johnson tells the two aids who didn't speak, that they are to escort Anjie down to her office in five minutes or so. "Give them a few minutes and then bring her down," she ordered, leaving briskly.

Goldman and Fine are standing in the doorway of the little office. "I can't believe this is happening," Goldman says. "Anjie is definitely not that woman. How can people make a mistake like that?"

133

"Maybe it is not a mistake," Harry says. "Maybe they are doing it on purpose."

"Let me go down there and talk with the sheriff. Maybe we can get to the bottom of this thing," Anjie says, confidently. "I just know this can't be happening."

Johnson's office is the office of a chief executive with expensive furniture and decorations. She has only one photo on her desk, that of a young woman. She sees Anjie's interest in the photo and explains, "My former companion," she says. "We were together for six months. I lost her in an auto accident."

Unsure what to say, Anjie ignored the reference to the sheriff's companion. "Am I under arrest?"

"No, you will be free to go. But I want to talk with you, man to man, so to speak, before this gets more serious for you. Frankly, we do not know what happened to Cleveland. As far as we are aware, a crime has not been committed. But then again, maybe he was abducted against his will. Men and women walk away from old folks' homes all the time. We get reports of missing patients just about every week. In most instances, they are found walking along the street, incoherent, confused, hungry and cold. No such luck with Cleveland. At some point, Ms de la Houssaye, this is going to be classified as a possible crime, and at that point, you are under suspicion for involvement in it. It would be helpful to me and to you-if you told me what your involvement is, so far."

Anjie liked Johnson. She admired her for her achievement, of course, but beyond that, she seemed a thoroughly professional person. She wondered to herself, could Johnson have been so bold about a female companion in the FBI? Probably not, she concluded. She was attractive and very feminine to have a traditionally male job. Anjie told her she looked like Cheryl Ladd did when she was Johnson's age. Johnson smiled. "And you are a dead-ringer for Madeline Stowe," Johnson said.

Anjie smiled and nodded agreement. "I've heard that before. It pleases me," she said. Johnson had put Angie at ease. Anjie trusted her. She decided to tell her the story, including the details about the law firm and Goldman. "In addition to the items relating to the inventions, I also inherited a very valuable piece of property in San Diego, at Rancho Santa Fe—a vacant lot. My Realtor listed it for $2-million. This was my incentive to come down here, to see the property. It belonged to my Uncle Moreau."

Johnson said she was very familiar with that area, that when she was with the FBI, her office was located there. Anjie explained where the vacant lot is located. "I know that property. I often wondered why there was not some commercial business there. I heard once that the property was tied up in litigation with heirs suing each other, that sort of thing. I had no idea it was owned all this time by a Canadian, who didn't even live in this area."

"It was a great surprise to me. I didn't know anything about it until a couple of days before leaving British Columbia for PEI. Even

135

then, I did not expect very much. It was described as a vacant lot, and it didn't sound like it was very valuable. When I came down here, I met the Realtor the law firm had hired to get an appraisal, and she said to list it for that amount, so I did."

"Who is the Realtor?"

"The Realtor? I have it here in my purse." She digs down in the wallet, removing a business card. She hands it to Johnson.

"Do you mind if I keep this?"

"No, I have the contact information on the listing documents," Anjie says.

"About these inventions you told me about. Do you have that diary with you?"

"Yes."

"Don't you think that should be in a safe place?"

"Yes."

"Call me when you have it in your hands. I'll send a car out to pick it up. We'll put it in our safe, until you leave. Also, what about the other stuff? Are you sure it is all secure?"

"Goldman took the drawings; I imagine they are at his apartment in PEI. The parts are still in the storage unit. I have similar documents at my home in a trunk. I have had this stuff for years but never bothered to know what it was." Anjie told Johnson she had become suspicious of the firm, and perhaps, Goldman—that she met with an FBI agent and in the same place, an Interpol agent. Johnson said she knew both men, and that they were good, reliable and honest people. "I'm really glad to hear that!," Anjie said.

"When you leave here, say nothing to Goldman or your minister friend about this conversation. Just tell them that we talked, and that you thought I was going to find Cleveland, or at least determine whether he left of his own volition or not. Let it go at that," she advised. "I'm worried about you, Ms de la Houssaye." She paused a moment and then asked, "Are either of these two men lovers?"

"No. I am not intimate with either of them," she said.

"Good. Sometimes that can cloud your judgment. About the FBI, this looks very good for you, that you took that step. It means you have the same concerns that I have. About those crutches, Ms de la Houssaye, I did some checking on you, and apparently you are quiet a success story."

"So are you, apparently—by the way, call me Anjie."

"You are a role model for others, that is for sure," Johnson said, pointing to a notebook computer on her desk. "I looked you up on the Internet and was surprised to see so many newspaper stories about you. I just wish that we had met under pleasant circumstances, instead of this messy investigation," Johnson shrugged.

"Write down all your contact numbers, address, and give it to me before you leave-"

"-I don't know them. I am staying at a condo belonging to a friend of Harry's," Anjie said, adding "Thank you for the way you are handling this. Actually, you are the role model for women. All I did was try to get better."

"And you did it!," Johnson said, triumphantly.

Johnson comes around the desk and sits on the edge of it near Anjie. She hands her a card. Call me when you get to the condo with all the numbers. AND if anything unusual happens at all, you call me," she says. "I don't want anything to happen to you."

"I'm glad. I don't want anything to happen to me, either! But what about those employees who identified me?"

"I am going to look into their backgrounds, to see what is there, if anything. You are in a very high stakes game right now, Anjie, and money is probably the least of worries for the people manipulating this thing. I want you to call me tomorrow, even if you don't hear from me." She gets up off the desk, extending her hands to Anjie for assistance. "One more thing, tell those guys absolutely nothing about this conversation. It's important that you listen to me," she smiled.

Accepting Johnson's assistance, she raised herself up out of the chair. "I got it. Thank you. If anyone can solve this puzzle, it's you. I just feel that way," Anjie said.

"I will do everything I can," Johnson promised.

———

Automobiles and trucks are filling the midsummer air with sounds of exhaust and engine roars. Outlying neighborhoods that can be seen from the freeway are evidence of postwar construction as these were among the first tracts built after the war. "I thought I would take you home a different way, so you can at least say you saw something while you were here," Harry said. Anjie smiled.

Finally, after what seemed to be endless traffic, they reach Hollywood Boulevard. Before long they are at the intersection of Hollywood and Vine, the streets of dreams and legends. They pass the Egyptian Theater and then Grauman's Chinese Theater. "I read not very long ago that a company of psychics claimed to have located ghosts in these old theaters," Anjie said.

"Ghosts? I don't believe in ghosts," he said. "But who doesn't like Hollywood? I mean the movies are a part of our lives. We pay to see them, even knowing that what we see is all made up, and that the actors are pretending to be people they are not; but yet, we are fascinated and go," he says.

"That's why we go. It is all escapism," she sighed. "Look there— a whole bus load of tourists getting out just to go walking down that street!"

There were only a few questions from Harry about the time Anjie spent with Johnson. Herb was visibly dazed that she shook him off, refusing to discuss the meeting, except to say that it was pleasant, and that the sheriff promised to find what happened to Cleveland and Gertrude Milhaus. Hurriedly, Anjie left in the protection of Harry.

"You don't have to tell me anything," Harry said. "I am here for you. As for GOLD-MAN, I don't like him AND I do not trust him! It is up to you to decide how to handle your business. Now that you are a millionaire, all sorts of people will be clinging to you," he said.

He's right, Anjie thought. Now that she had money or at least the prospects of getting money, she would acquire new friends, she didn't doubt that at all. But Anjie is a realist, not about to count her chickens before she sees them. Until that property is sold, and she has the check in her hands, she is going to be very cautious about money.

As for Goldman, she is thinking she cannot afford to just blow him off—he has the drawings and plans from the storage unit and until she gets them back, she must not split with him to the point where they part on unfriendly terms. "Give me your cell phone," Anjie orders, "please. I'm thinking I better call Herb. I don't want him so angry with me that he leaves. He has those drawings, I have to be very careful about what happens between us until I get those drawings back."

Harry removes the phone from his side jacket pocket, handing it to Anjie. "Be careful, but I guess you're right," he said. "We're stopping up here at a really great restaurant. We're in no hurry to get back to La Jolla tonight. Are we?"

Anjie nodded agreement.

12

Wind is blowing rain against the windows of the room while lightning flashes outside. Men are in the bedroom looking, talking and dusting. Uniformed police are on the porch out of the rain, smoking and talking. A police vehicle idles with flashing lights. On a cot in the bedroom of the small house lies the fully clothed body of Dr. Cyrus Cleveland. A man and a woman are standing over him. "Transport him to the morgue, there is nothing more we can do here. There are no external signs that I can see of any trauma. He looks like he died of natural causes," the man says to the woman; she agrees. The woman throws a sheet up over his body. "I am estimating that he is dead about 12 hours," he says. "He is a John Doe." They both leave the room.

It's June and it rains a lot in New Orleans. Natives don't seem to mind, they even welcome it as a relief from the heat. This small house does not have air conditioning or very much furniture. There is an ice chest on the floor near the bed with the cool remains of what was ice, and a single bottle of Abita Springs water. An opened package of processed ham lays at the bottom of the chest. An opened box of crackers is next to it. There is no refrigerator or stove, but there is a coffee pot with a half filled bag of French Market Coffee and Chicory. There is one used paper cup with a little coffee and a cigarette butt.

"We have a few things here, not much," Sgt. Rodney Delacroix says, "wrap this stuff up, just in case this is not a natural cause case." The plain-clothes policeman, a young man, obviously wishing he were somewhere else, dutifully places the items in baggies. Delacroix, a 12-year veteran, has seen many crime scenes in his day. "This all looks benign but that is suspicious in itself; this old guy is well-dressed and appears in good physical condition. What would he be doing in a rat-hole like this?" No one responds.

"There is nothing in the bathroom of a personal nature, either," Sarge, a young officer says. "Nothing but a role of toilet paper."

"Bag it!" Delacroix barks, grinning.

The house is only three rooms on lower Chartres Street built seventy or eighty years ago; it is now abandoned. It is one of the old French style 'shotgun' houses that are still common in New Orleans. In some sections of the city, close to the French Quarter, young persons are buying up places like this to tear down, so they can build a new house that looks old, a trend that appears to be catching on all over the historical part of the city.

142

The police work here is grunt work. The property belongs or belonged to someone, and that must be determined; but if that doesn't lead to anywhere, they will have to rely on what they can get through forensics. But at this point there is no homicide investigation, because there is the preliminary belief that the old man died of natural causes. As to why he is in a place like this, that may not ever be known. It could be that the old man died somewhere else and was brought here, the perpetrators thinking he would not be found. If it were not for a routine inspection scheduled to post a notice that the property was subject to being destroyed by the city, he may not have been found while he was still recognizable.

The body leaves and so do the police, but first they string yellow tape over the front porch to show what is left of a neighborhood that the house is a crime scene. Chartres is just one street in a grid of narrow one-way streets. It runs from Canal Street all the way through the French Quarter. This house is located near the end of the street opposite an abandoned lumberyard.

―――――

Tony Pecoro and Bob Simpson are in San Diego on the yacht "Prescription." They are meeting with Turner von Atziger, Herb Goldman and the private detective, Charles. Pecoro and Simpson are visibly aggravated, speaking in loud voices. Charles is cowering down in a chair with Simpson standing over him. "Those fuck ups you hired

143

to get Cleveland out of here really screwed up. They took the money you gave them and killed the old man. Do you realize what this does? The guy is dead. Now we will never know what he knew about that cancer cure," Simpson yells. Charles stares down at the floor.

"It is only because one of them called me that we even know they did this. He is scared and says the other two forced him into it," Charles says. "What can I do? I've used these people before without a problem-"

"-Yea but it did not involve big money. You gave them $50,000 to take the guy away. They should have made him as comfortable as possible, following our plan by telling him that if he cooperated, nothing would happen to him. But instead, they throw the guy in a van and drive him all the way to New Orleans to kill him," Pecoro yells.

"If it means anything," Charles says, "Lucy said that the guy was killed accidentally. Big Mike got tired of the old guy refusing to cooperate, and was going to show him what could happen. He put a baggie around his head to cut off his breathing for a few minutes but, unfortunately, his death was almost immediate."

"Charles, you're finished," Simpson says. "Finished."

Pecoro pulls a .357 Magnum from his jacket pocket and without a word, fires one bullet into Charles' head. For some reason none of them understood, there was very little blood, only a few drops dripping down his forehead.

"I never signed up for this," Goldman says. "This has all gone too far. This was a simple operation that is now out of control. Now two people are dead." Goldman is pacing the floor, but his eyes follow Pecoro's every move.

"Goldman, part of this problem is yours. All you had to do was get into the woman's pants to gain her cooperation and trust, follow her back to British Columbia and gather up the other documents she has on this Rife invention. Then you were through but no, you couldn't even do that-"

"-I tried. The woman is a born again Christian. For God's sake, I'm Jewish. This whole plan was flawed from the beginning."

"Maybe, but Mr. Loebel bet this whole project on the idea that you could make her do what was needed, but you did not execute your end," Simpson said. "Charles is dead because he didn't complete his assignment."

"Is that a warning? Don't do anything foolish, I have the engineering notes and drawings hidden where no one will ever find them," Goldman says, impatiently. "Besides, if I am dead, how can the firm explain that vacant lot de la Houssaye supposedly inherited? You need me to blame for that 'mistake'. Don't forget it."

Pecoro drops the gun back in his pocket. "Calm down. We need to regroup. We're all in this together, and now we need to figure out where we go from here."

Turner von Atziger, who had been sitting quietly and undisturbed by the killing of Charles on his yacht, stands up. "I will tell you guys one thing, and it is something you better remember. I put this whole deal together with the consortium—they want these instruments or whatever they are that Rife invented. They want them reconstructed to see if they work, and if that doesn't happen, they are not going to be happy that we are spending all of this money and screwing up all over the place. You still have the woman. Make the best of that. Get her to cooperate, if you can't, kill her. We don't have much time to waste on this. IF the plan to retrieve all the possible parts, drawings, and whatever expertise is left alive does not work-and it appears now it is danger of not working-then the only other option is to gather it all up. Give it to me to deliver to my associates. They will be satisfied knowing they have all of it, and that it can't be assembled. Once that is done, the firm comes into a gush of money and that's what we all share."

"What about Goldman?" Simpson asked. "What do we do with him?"

"Go home. If we succeeded today, two persons who saw Cleveland leave with her and a strange man identified De la Houssaye. When Cleveland's death is known, she will be held as a suspect. While she is tied up in deep do-do down here, we will be up in British Columbia going through her underwear draws," Pecoro grinned.

Everyone agrees.

Herb Goldman and Anjie are sitting at a table drinking coffee. Anjie has finished her breakfast but Herb has not touched his. He appears to be nervous. The waitress lays a check on the table, smiles and walks away. Herb stares at his uneaten food.

"Herb, I'm sorry this did not work out for us. I regret that you must go back to PEI, while this is all still unsettled. I do want you to promise me that you will take those drawings and notes from wherever you have them, and keep them safe for me," Anjie said.

"I can't get rid of this awful feeling that I am leaving you here with more problems than we came with." He picks up the bill and walks over to the cashier where he pays it. Anjie follows him. For a very brief moment, Herb looks intently into Anjie's eyes; they scare him. She is confident, showing no signs of the worry that he himself has. They make their way outside the restaurant where Wolfgang is waiting to drive Herb to the airport. Harry Fine is sitting in the limo next to Wolfgang, waiting for Anjie.

"Get yourself a good lawyer. Those ID's made by those nursing home employees mean absolutely nothing. They prove nothing, but you need representation," he says. "I'm going to miss you."

They hug briefly. Harry exits the limousine, wishing Herb a safe trip. As they drive away, Harry wonders aloud whether Herb is really leaving. "Why don't we go out there to see if he makes that flight?," Harry asked.

"For a Christian man of God, you are very untrusting," Anjie retorted. "Let's go for a ride and then do a little shopping in La Jolla. Frankly, I don't care if he gets on that plane or not."

———

A pile of garments lay dirty in the middle of the floor in the living room. Laura is bending over wearing only a crimson red sweatshirt with the name "Harvard University" written across it. She is surprised that from under the pile she has retrieved a purse, and one shoe. She throws them back. Impatiently, finally, she chooses a pair of panties. She slides them on. The cell phone rings on the table next to a left over pizza. It is Herb Goldman.

"I handled everything for you with Tony Pecoro. He wired the funds you requested."

"All of it?" she asked, still rummaging through the pile.

"All of it. He said for you to stay put, in case de la Houssaye tries to contact you about that property. If you have any contact with her at all, he wants to know about it. Do you understand, Laura?"

"Sure, I understand. There is nothing to worry about. That dumb bitch will never know what hit her. I don't expect to hear from her again very soon, but I am standing by like I agreed, as long as the money is in the bank," she said. She matches a pair of nylons while she listens.

"Don't fuck up, Laura, I hate to tell you what can happen, if you do," he said.

"You don't have to spoon feed me. This is not my first rodeo," she says, sarcastically.

"Stay in character so that you don't screw up. BE SUDSY LANAHAN at all times," he suggested.

"Why don't you come over to see 'Sudsy' for yourself?"

"Can't- I am on my way back to Canada," he said.

"Stay in touch. Right now I am on my way to the bank to see if that money is there." She hangs up, still throwing garments around the room.

13

The room is pitch black. Sitting on the edge of the bed is Anjie. She is breathing heavy. Suddenly the door whips open, flooding the room with light. "Anjie, did you call me?"

Anjie nods her head negatively. "I had a bad dream, I guess. I woke up in a cold sweat," she explains. "I'll be OK but I think I am going to stay awake for now. What time is it?"

"It is nearly five." Harry is wearing short pants and a t-shirt. He sits down next to Anjie, wrapping one arm around her. "Are you sure you are OK?"

"Yes. I'm sorry, but I guess I called out during the dream. Funny thing is that I don't even remember what it was about," she chuckled. "Please excuse me a few minutes while I get dressed."

"Good idea. We can then watch the sun rise together over the ocean," he said. "I'll make some coffee." He leaves the room.

On the balcony with their coffee, they both watch as the bright orange glow of the sun first appears and then moves gradually across the sky. "Anjie, I want to see that property you inherited while I am here. Why don't we ride out there later?"

"Great! Maybe seeing all that money laying there in the form of mud and grass will cheer me up," she says, adding, "I still feel a little like I have cobwebs in my head. Waking up like that is probably not good for your health."

Harry laughs. "You'll be alright. After all you've been through, I am not surprised that you have bad dreams. That stuff at the sheriff's office has to upset you. What a bummer," he says, pouring more coffee into Anjie's cup. "I just can't believe those people at that nursing home."

"I trust that it will all work out. The sheriff believes me, I'm sure of that. Any way, she said herself, even with the identification, there is nothing they can do to me, as there is no evidence whatsoever that anything has happened to Cleveland or that if it did, that I know anything about it," she says, confidently. "Besides, I trust Sheriff Johnson."

"We'll have breakfast here, then take that ride to see the property," she says. "I just have trouble believing that one day I will have nearly $2-million in cash. God is too good to me."

"God is looking out for you. He has for many years," Herb says, kissing her on her forehead. "Your life is precious to us all."

———

A tractor, pulling a trailer loaded with a large farm machine, slowly makes its way down the narrow two lane road under a majestic, cloud-filled sky. Harry patiently follows the tractor, frequently changing gears as the engine of the Porsche roars its displeasure at having to travel below 40 miles per hour. Anjie is enjoying the countryside.

"I didn't know there are places left in southern California like this," she sighs, "it is really beautiful out here. I'm enjoying this scenic route you chose."

Harry says nothing. He is impatiently pulling out and back in, waiting for an opportunity to pass the tractor. "We are only five miles from the entrance to the freeway. I will get back on it, so that we can get to Rancho Santa Fe sometime today," he laughed.

Harry is being a friend. He is making no demands of Anjie. Even though he is tender and caring with her, he is not aggressive in any way. Anjie is not sure whether she likes that or not. In the back of her mind, she is hoping for romance. She is thinking that her disability is more of a problem than she admits.

"Harry, will you tell me the truth, if I ask you a question?"

"Of course."

"Why do you think it is that men compliment me endlessly on my appearance, and resemblance to Madcline Stowe, but do nothing to have a relationship with me? Is it my disability?"

"Wow! What a question? I think that any man who knows you, well - they are not going to even think about that disability. They are going to love you for whom you are. I'm certain of that."

"Then why haven't they?"

"How many men do you know, Anjie?" He then answers his own question. "You don't get out much back home. You spend all your time at that newspaper, and other than church gatherings, and volunteer work, how do you get out to meet men?"

"I don't know a lot of men but the men I do know, they have no interest in me, and yet they tell me repeatedly how beautiful I am," she says.

"I think you are beautiful. I've told you that many times; but you do not seem to pay attention. You thank me or say nothing but smile. If you do that every time a man compliments you, you are not going to get much follow up-"

"-In other words, I turn them off," she shrugs.

"You just do not reciprocate interest, Anjie. Maybe you are not ready for a serious relationship."

"What about you?"

He laughs. "I've heard the rumors that some people think I'm gay. I'm NOT gay. Believe me, being gay in a NFL locker room, that is something I would have to see! No, I am not gay. Before coming to the Lord, I had many women, Anjie. I am ashamed to tell you about it. I've done it all. But now, I am just waiting for the right person to come along. When I meet her, I am going to marry her!," he says, confidently.

Up until the time they exit the freeway, they do not speak. Anjie feels better, but she realizes she did not get an answer. She will have to do what Harry is doing-wait until that right person comes along.

"This is one of the main streets. You should be seeing a Mexican restaurant with a large sombrero as a sign. The property is across the street from the restaurant, next to a small medical building."

"There it is," he says, enthusiastically. "I can't wait to see what $2-million of dirt looks like!"

She points to it as they approach. "Looks like there are some men walking around on the lot," she says. "I wonder what that is all about?"

"Could be they are appraising it for the real estate listing. Or who knows? Maybe the Realtor already has a prospect for it," he said. He drives the car up to the corner and then backs in out of the way of the pedestrian lane, and the 'Do Not Park' sign. "Let's see what they are doing."

Anjie is excited. "Dare I feel so optimistic that this property is going to sell this fast?" Helping her from the car, Harry nods his head yes.

There are four men in suits walking about and talking. There are two men who are putting up stakes and running line from one to the other. Herb and Anjie approach the men who are looking at an architectural rendering, held by one of the men. The drawing is of a national drug store chain of retailers.

"Hi, I am Harry Fine. This is Anjie de la Houssaye. What are you guys doing?"

"What? Who are you?," the older man asked.

"Sorry. I am a friend of Anjie's-"

"-I own this property; it is for sale. We passed by, saw you out here, and thought we would stop to see what is going on-"

The men stare at each other, obviously confused. "Lady, I don't know who you are. Our company has been negotiating with the owners of this property for three years, while the estate of the owner was in succession. We bought it, finally, for $6.5 million. We are putting up a drive- through pharmacy here!"

Harry extends his arm up, stopping Anjie from saying anything. "How is that possible? Anjie inherited this property from her uncle. She just listed it for sale this week-"

"-I don't know who you folks are," the well-dressed, older man says threateningly, "but you are on the wrong property. The owners are all relatives of the person who died; they have been fighting over the percentages of the proceeds for years. They finally settled. Nearly all of them live in Hawaii. Now who this woman is or what she thinks she owns, that is something else entirely."

Anjie is shaken. Suddenly, she falls to the ground. Harry picks her up; he carries her to the Porsche. One of the men follows with her crutches. "Sorry, buddy, but this is some sort of tragic mistake."

Harry fits Anjie in the car, begging her to wake up. Finally, she does. "I dropped. I felt the blood leaving my body. It is a strange feeling, one that I've not had in a very long time. As for this situation here, I think we better go to the Realtor to find out what this is all about."

Anjie removes a file from her attaché. "They are located at 1515 Palm Springs Drive. Here is their phone number. Call them for directions," she says, handing the file over to Herb. He dials the number and returns the file.

In less than three minutes, they are in the parking lot of the real estate company. En route there, Anjie said nothing. Harry prayed there was some sort of mistake. The receptionist is an attractive woman in her twenties, well dressed and personable. "Do you have someone in mind that you want to see?"

"Yes," Anjie replied, "Sudsy Lanahan, the Realtor who listed my property."

"Just a moment." The young woman turns away and into an office nearby. A man in his fifties emerges. He is short, overweight and bald. He doesn't look like a Realtor. The young woman presents the man. "This is Mr. O'Reilly," she says. "He is our office manager. He will assist you." She goes away.

"How may I be of service?," O'Reilly asked. He is smiling and friendly.

"We want to see Sudsy Lanahan," Anjie says, emphatically.

"We do not have anyone by that name in any position. Are you sure you are in the right place?"

Anjie withdraws the listing agreement from her attaché. She hands it to O'Reilly. "It is the standard listing form we all use but wait, we just sold this property listed here, after very difficult negotiations. What is this supposed to be?"

At this point, Harry realizes that Anjie has been scammed. "This woman who claimed she worked for you, listed this property for sale for $2-million. Anjie here was told by her attorneys she inherited it, and even has the papers on it."

"What did this woman look like?"

"A slut—I'm sorry, I didn't mean that. She was young, very sexy and provocatively dressed. Extremely flirtatious."

O'Reilly laughed. "I hate to tell you this, but that could be any number of women we have working as agents for us. If I were you, I would go to a lawyer to get this handled. That form is legitimate but this Lanahan didn't list any property, and she does not work for us. I'm sorry."

"You're sorry? Believe me," Anjie says, "you don't know what it means to be sorry. My whole future is changed. I wake up and find that I am back where I started," she says. "I'm disgusted and sad. I want to find out why this was done and who did it," she tells Harry. "Let's go see the sheriff."

14

"First, let me say that I'm a very ordinary person. My profession is that of journalist. A small market journalist, an editor really, of the only paper in a city of 8,000. I had a terrible accident when I was twelve years old; I was told I would never walk again. You can see that through monumental effort, God's help and rehabilitation that I can walk and, truthfully, get along pretty well. There is absolutely nothing in my life up until this point, to suggest that I should be the subject of a dreadful plot of some kind that has engulfed my life, and invaded it to the point where it is all that is on my mind. Months ago I was advised by the law firm in PEI that I had an inheritance from my Uncle Andre Moreau. I was told there was practically no money, but there was a rooming house in PEI that had no mortgage or liens, and was rented most of the time.

"Property in San Diego was not mentioned until shortly before I was due to leave my home for Charlottetown. There was no reference to the value of it. I was told there is a vacant lot; where I'm from, a lot is vacant because it has no useful purpose; I assumed this was the case in San Diego," Anjie pauses to take a sip of bottled water.

"Go on, please, Anjie," the sheriff urged. "Go on."

"Herb Goldman was assigned my file when another lawyer who had been handling it resigned from the firm. I liked Herb from the first moment of meeting him. He is bright and thorough. I trusted him. He produced a key to a storage unit in Charlottetown that he said he did not know about until the day before I arrived. We agreed to go there together to see what was in it. This is where we found the old newspaper clips, the schematic drawings and engineering notes, and an estimated 6,000 parts of instruments along with the diary. You have the diary, so you know what it is about.

"This man by the name of Royal Rife lived in San Diego with his wife of Chinese descent. Rife's father-in-law was very wealthy, providing huge sums of money for him to do his research. During this period, eventually, after years of trial and error, Rife developed the most powerful microscope in the world. This microscope enabled him to see germs that, he said, caused diseases. He got the idea that if he electrocuted these germs, that he could cure diseases without drugs. You know the rest of what happened to him and his inventions, and it was not good," Anjie says, emphatically.

"Goldman and I decided to come to San Diego. Well, he knew I wanted to come to view the vacant lot he said I inherited. I need cash, so whatever its value is, I intended to sell it, keeping the income producing property at PEI. Goldman suggested that he could join me here, and that together we could look into this Rife invention thing, and see if we could locate Dr. Cleveland, who is mentioned quite often in that diary. So this is what we did, and now I am sitting here in your office, and, truthfully, I do not have a clue any more as to what is going on." Anjie is holding back tears as well as she can. "Sheriff, I don't know what to do next."

Johnson comes from behind the desk. She sits next to Anjie. She comforts her. "Call me Cherie, that is what my friends call me," she says calmly. "Don't worry, I will help you get this unraveled."

"A few minutes ago we left the real estate office, where the woman who said she listed this San Diego property worked. We were told she did not work there, and this property was sold for $6-million, following protracted negotiations with a drug store chain. We had already heard that because we stopped by at the site, and men were there doing engineering and planning. They thought I was some sort of nut when I told them I owned the property," Anjie said, tearfully. She tries a grin: "I guess I am a nut to believe all this."

"I planned to investigate this real estate deal and agent when you gave me the woman's business card. In fact, I have someone on it right now. It didn't sound right to me, frankly, because I know that property is in succession for years; also, I know it is worth a lot more than $2-million," the sheriff says, confidently. "Our attorneys are also checking on it, to see who the previous owners were. We'll know in a short while."

Cherie Johnson is not wearing her sheriff's uniform today. Instead, she is wearing a blue business suit. She is a natural blonde who wears her hair short. Anjie wondered how much more attractive Cherie would look, if she allowed her hair to reach her shoulders. She likes Cherie and it is obvious Cherie likes Anjie. Anjie is a strong-willed person who has overcome many obstacles in the course of beating her handicap. But this situation has her teary and sad. She finds that Cherie has strength she is drawing on to help relieve her pain.

"I tried calling your Mr. Goldman this morning on his cell phone and at the office in PEI. He did not answer the phone, and the office claims he has not arrived from California. According to the airline, he was on the plane to New Brunswick, so we have to assume he arrived. Either his office is lying or he has not shown up yet."

"What did you want with him?"

"I wanted to ask him who did the title search on this San Diego property."

"Oh, I guess we know now. But what I don't know is why he did this to me? There is no gain in it for him or the law firm, from what I can tell," Anjie said.

"Why go through the trouble to convince me I have property here, then hire someone to act as if they are a real estate agent? How do they profit from this?"

"I can't answer those questions now. We can guess but we do not know. All we know is that he or someone else set up an elaborate scheme to make you think you owned this property, and that you would be rich when it was sold."

The buzzer sounds. "Excuse me, let me take this call." Johnson reaches over the desk; she hits a button. "I said I did not want to be disturbed."

"Take it, sheriff. It is a police detective in New Orleans. He is talking about a connection on a case," the young woman on the other end says, persuading Johnson to disconnect without a word. She picks up the phone.

"Sheriff Johnson," she says, authoritatively, reaching for a pen and pad.

"Sheriff, this is Det. Sgt. Delacroix in New Orleans. We have a John Doe here that resembles one of your missing persons. The name on your alert is Dr. Cyrus Cleveland," he says.

Johnson turns to Anjie, excitedly. "Just a minute, allow me to put you on the speaker. Go ahead-"

"Like I said, your alert states you are looking for a man in his seventies by the name of Cyrus Cleveland. We have a dead John Doe here that fits that description."

"Certainly. How did he die?"

"Appears to be natural causes," he says. "We found him in a rundown old shack off the French Quarter. The surroundings arc suspicious, but the coroner tells us there are no signs of any trauma or internal injuries. No drugs were found in his body that could have killed him, either. He is old and the coroner says he just stopped breathing."

"He stopped breathing? Why did he find this shack to die-in?"

"I have no idea about that. We speculate that someone took him there. Maybe his death is very inconvenient for someone. Who knows? But the report is definite. Natural causes."

"Thank you, Detective. I appreciate your good work. Please return the body to us at our expense. Hold on I will connect you with our coordinator." Johnson hits a number and someone answers. "Take this call," she says.

"You heard. Cleveland is dead but supposedly of natural causes. Whoever it was picked the old guy up in San Diego County to take him all the way to New Orleans. You know when he left that home that he had no idea he was leaving town. He didn't take one pair of trousers, underwear or even a shirt, as far as we can tell. God, I wish I knew why-"

"-You can bet it has something to do with the Rife inventions and my possession of it. Cleveland may have been able to direct the reassembling of it. Now we will never know," Anjie says, sadly.

"Know what?"

"If the cure for diseases can be reassembled."

There is a pause while both women regain their composures. "I know, let's take a break. Do you like Chinese food? I know a great place that is only a few blocks from here. We can talk some more while we are out."

"I would like that but Harry Fine is in the room waiting for me-"

"-Oh no, I had him sent away. The deputy told him to leave his numbers that we'd call him when we are ready for him to pick you up. I knew this might take most of the day," she said.

"Good. I don't feel like re-living all of this right now with Harry," Anjie said.

A group of men, mostly construction workers, whistle and make obscene gestures and sounds as Anjie and Cherie enter the Chinese restaurant. Anjie ignores them but Cherie flips them a birdie. Anjie laughs. "If only they knew you were the sheriff," she says, "I have a feeling we would have gotten a more gentlemanly greeting."

Only three or four people are sitting at tables. "This place is new and great but people haven't discovered it yet," Cherie explains. "We don't have to stay here. We can carry it to my place, I live only a few blocks from here."

Their order is quickly ready. The Chinese man at the window taking the orders says he added a few things he wanted them to try. They thank him and leave. This time the men are too busy to worry them.

The view of the mountains from the house is extraordinary. Anjie stands at a window looking down at a great pool and cabana. An Asian woman about 55 greeted them at the door and then prepared the food for serving. Cherie changed into a pair of genes and a halter. "I hope you make yourself at home, Anjie. I changed into something more comfortable. If you would like to do the same, I am certain I have clothes that will fit you perfectly."

Anjie thanks her but declines the offer.

The Asian woman serves the food and then Cherie dismisses her. "Thank you Shakila. If we need you again we will call you."

Cherie sees Anjie's awe over the expensive house in an even more expensive neighborhood. She volunteers to Anjie that the house is inherited from her father who was quite wealthy. "He made a lot of money. Unfortunately, he died too young," Cherie said, sadly.

Cherie's cell phone rings. She looks at the number on the display panel. "We want to take this one," she says to Anjie, clicking on the speaker feature. "Hello, Roger, what did you find out?"

"The property was once owned by Andre Moreau but it was foreclosed many years ago when the most recent owner acquired it from the bank for the unbelievable sum of $600,000," he said. "So, you are right, it was in the family at one point," he says.

"Thank you, Roger, that is all I need for now. If Harriet is there, ask her if she retrieved any financial information on Dr. Cyrus Cleveland." Roger says nothing but in a few seconds, Harriet Wilson, another lawyer working in the sheriff's office, is on the line.

"Sheriff, the nursing home had a complete financial package on Cleveland, also, the name of his attorney. I called the attorney. He told me that Cleveland is worth about $1-million, mostly in cash and securities. I told him he is missing and asked him to check the accounts to see if any money is being moved. He pulled the accounts up on the Internet and guess what? No money has been withdrawn since Cleveland left the home. NOT ONE CENT."

"Harriet, thank you. I will talk to you later."

"Anjie, you heard the conversations. The fact that no money is being used from Cleveland's accounts proves that he was not taken for money, or that he did leave voluntarily on his own volition. If it was anything else, the funds would be tapped," she said, serving Anjie and then herself from the vegetable tray.

"Oh, eat that—it is extraordinary," Cherie says, pointing to a cluster of broccoli mixed with other vegetables.

"I still haven't heard from the guys I sent out to investigate the so-called real estate agent who listed the property, Sudsy Lanahan. I am hoping they find her. If they do, we will know then why that scam was concocted."

"God, you really have a job—you were with the FBI and now you run this big organization. I don't know how you do it," Anjie said, admiring Cherie. "You seem to have a handle on every little detail."

"I could handle it much better if I had someone like you handling my contacts with the media," she said.

Anjie said nothing but she smiled warmly.

———

"Finding the woman was not that difficult once we knew she was driving a rented Mercedes sports coupe. We gave the description Ms de la Houssaye gave the department and bingo! We went to the apartment where she was staying. She wasn't there, so we waited down the block. When the Mercedes showed up, so did we!," said Deputy Bill Miller. "She was shaken up, you can believe that. We asked her if we could search her car and belongings and she said yes. We found $50,000 in mixed bills. She had just picked it up from a bank. Joel Watkins is down at the bank now finding out who sent it," he said.

"Excellent! You guys did great work. Great!"

Anjie is shocked. "I can't believe you found her so quickly. Amazing."

"Who do you think gave her that money?"

"The firm is my guess," Anjie said "or maybe Goldman for the firm."

A few minutes later, Joel Watkins calls into the office to speak with Deputy Miller. Miller tells him to go directly to the sheriff that she is waiting to hear from him. The story is that the money was sent from Latvia from a numbered account. "There is no way to know unless the suspect tells us," he says.

"She is in headquarters in a holding cell. You get back here and question her with Miller. Keep me informed," the sheriff says.

"We can't keep her very long without charging her and right now, we don't have any thing to charge her with," Cherie says. "Nothing!"

"What about the phony real estate listing?"

"Well, we might be able to stretch that into a misdemeanor but it wont hold up. She could always say it was a joke. Or she could blame it on Goldman. You didn't give her any money, did you?"

"No."

The sheriff's secretary enters carrying a note. She hands it to Cherie and waits for a response. "Verify this and then let me know," she says softly. "Verify it, for God's sake, verify it!"

She is visibly upset. She offers no explanation to Anjie. "Excuse me. I will be right back," she says. Cherie leaves the office through the same door as the secretary. She is gone five or more minutes. When she returns, her color is gone.

"Anjie, I just received some incredible news. It is verified by one of the partners of the firm at Price Edward Island and the Mounties. It is unbelievable but true: Herb Goldman is dead. He was driving from St. Johns in New Brunswick to PEI via the Confederation Bridge. He lost control of the car just as he crossed over and went off the road. There is a report from the Mounties that there was a considerable odor of alcohol."

Anjie is silent for a minute or so and then cries heartily. Cherie drops to one knee and puts her arms around her. Anjie allows her head to rest on Cherie's chest. She is distraught, confused and saddened by the news. "Am I responsible for all this that is happening around me?," she sobs.

"Absolutely not. You're a victim. You are responsible now only for your own safety," she whispers. Anjie let it out. You have a lot to deal with—"

"I am so happy you are here with me," she says. "So very happy."

Cherie buzzes for her secretary. When she enters, she gives her orders: "Call Rev. Harry Fine. Tell him that Ms de la Houssaye is staying in a safe place tonight and that he will hear from her at some point but not to worry."

The secretary glances down to see Anjie crying, and Cherie holding her. "Yes, mam," she says. "I'll call him."

"You're staying with me tonight," Cherie said.

"Thank you."

————

The office has no name on it. It is in the same suburban complex as the U.S. Post Office. Inside, the office is spacious but sparsely furnished. The walls are empty. No FBI seals or plaques, personal accommodations, photographs or certificates or degrees. Sheriff Johnson steps inside, somewhat unsure of herself, and looks at Special Agent Reese McCordell, seated behind a plan, metal desk. McCordell acknowledges Johnson by waving her in. Anjie follow her.

McCordell motions for them to sit down. "I read the 302 on file. Since then some preliminary investigative work was authorized outside of the Agent-in-Charge's Office downtown. We came up clean. We have no evidence of any wrongdoing in connection with the disappearance of Dr. Cleveland from the nursing home or the woman, Gertrude Milhaus. In fact, we cannot not even find anyone who can identify Milhaus or who admits to knowing her. We closed our files on these issues."

"You couldn't find even one person out of those persons listed in the directory with the surname Milhaus, who admit to knowing her?," Anjie asked.

"No. In fact, the only person who says there is someone by that name is you. By the way, we checked with Social Security, finding a record of a person by that name that has been deceased for about ten years. What do you make of that?," he asked, somewhat sarcastically.

"Agent McCordell, I have a report from New Orleans that Cleveland was found dead in some slum dwelling and the police over there are claiming he died of natural causes. We have one dead end after the other."

McCordell agrees, "You are right and this is why we closed our files. As for Mr. Goldman, we checked him out and he is also clean. There were some questions about his friendship with Turner von Atziger, an international money merchant in the pharmaceutical industry, but nothing has come of it. Interpol was actually conducting an investigation of von Atziger but no longer. They came up clean, also."

"What did they think he did?," asked Anjie.

"Money laundering. There is a lot of smoke but after two years of investigating, they came up with nothing."

Cherie rises unexpectedly. "Thank you for your time. I'm sorry that you were not able to help us."

A trace of a smile shows up on McCordell's face. He walks over to the window and stares outside, and then quickly turns around. "Something has happened here but we don't know what it is, and probably never will."

The two women leave without a word.

15

In late June, lupines bloom on Prince Edward Island, adding to the scenic beauty that already includes unforgettable wooden churches, each one different but clean and surrounded by greenery. There seems to be a lighthouse in every part of the island inspiring anyone with a camera to start clicking. "I'm so glad you could come up during this time of year," Anjie says, "from now until early September, there is one special event after another. While we are here together we can take in as many as you want. If you like music, there are many live performances and dramas, too."

"You have a remarkable ability to accept what comes to you in life, Anjie. I respect that greatly. After all that has happened that is bad, you still see the positive side of life," Cherie says, leaning over to kiss her lightly on the cheek. "Thank you for inviting me."

Anjie and Cherie are riding in a rented, specially equipped Suburban. Anjie tells Cherie it is the same one she drove from St. Johns. "Where going to PEI National Park now. We can walk along the beaches, if we feel like it or go to Greenwich, a place where they have artifacts from the major cultures that have made up PEI over the centuries. Millions of potatoes are grown, as are blueberries and strawberries. Where else can you go where the farmers put their stuff out on the road with a sign and a box? You are on the honor system as to paying."

"What I want is lobster," Cherie says, excitedly. "I've read about lobsters in the east all of my life but in California we get those small lobsters from Australia. Did you make those reservations at Lobster on the Wharf at Charlottetown?"

"I did! I bet that when I go back with you to San Diego that if we try, we can find great lobsters there, also," Anjie says, smiling.

Cherie looks at Anjie intently. Anjie sees her. "What?"

"I'm so sorry that we did not solve this case and that you lost everything. Realistically, with Goldman dying, I didn't ever expect to see those drawings but when Rev. Fine called to tell you that the trunk in your basement at BC is missing, which sort of completed the insult. No one seems to know anything about any of this. A hopeless case, as far as law enforcement is concerned. No one gets charged with anything."

"It is not your fault or the FBI or Interpol or the Mounties. I realize now that what we were fighting is far too big, even for law enforcement. Is it any wonder that the pharmaceutical-medical complex prevented the Rife inventions from being exploited? No!

There is no way that a cure for diseases will ever be in use, unless it goes through them and is a drug."

Cherie rolls her head. "Still, it is wrong. The parts are gone from the storage unit-amazingly, no one has seen anything. And I couldn't even file a misdemeanor charge against that woman for scamming you in San Diego. She claimed the $50,000 was for other duties performed for the firm, not just that real estate gag. It is nonsense and ridiculous but with Goldman dead, we have no proof to the contrary. I am disappointed I couldn't even do that for you."

"At least Mr. Loebel let me keep the $50,000 as a sort of payment. I guess I was surprised when he blamed the whole property thing in San Diego on Goldman. You and I know that he had to know that Goldman didn't do that on his own," she said. "He claims that Goldman accepted the records from San Diego without checking them and that he did not do a title search."

"Tragically, there is never going to be a way to determine whether the Rife instruments could cure diseases or not. That's the way THEY want it, so that is the way it will be," Anjie said, obviously resigned to the facts.

"At least you have the diary for safe keeping. It is a great historical document. Perhaps you can write a book one day about all of this," Cherie says, cheerfully.

"I destroyed it. Who would believe a story like this?"

The End

174

ABOUT THE AUTHOR

R. E. PAYNE

The author is a director of two business graduate universities, Southern States University at Huntington Beach, California and Ashington University at Metairie, Louisiana (www.southernstatesuniversity.com and www.ashington university.com). He also serves as a Special Assistant to the Governor of the state of Louisiana. His memberships in professional organizations include the Chartered Institute of Professional Management, World Association for Online Education, Association for Supervision and Curriculum Development, American Evaluation Association and Canadian Association for Distance Education.

Payne is also the author of two non fiction books, "Caught in the Crossfire" (also a NBC-TV movie and "Above the Law, the hidden career of John Volz, USA." He is perhaps best known for his international best selling periodical "The Death of Brandon Lee: The Untold Story."

Payne's website is www.repayne.com.

Printed in the United States
16495LVS00005B/61